Recent Advances in

Histopathology
21

Recent Advances in Histopathology 20
Edited by DG Lowe & JCE Underwood

ISBN 1-85315-511-X

ISSN 0-0143 6953

Recent Advances in

Histopathology
21

Edited by

Massimo Pignatelli MD PhD FRCPath

Professor of Histopathology and Head of Department,
Department of Clinical Science South Bristol, University of Bristol, UK

James C. E. Underwood MD FRCP FMedSci FRCPath

Joseph Hunter Professor of Pathology, Academic Unit of Pathology,
University of Sheffield, Sheffield, UK

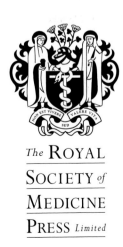

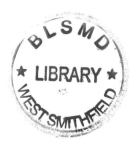

The ROYAL
SOCIETY *of*
MEDICINE
PRESS Limited

© 2005 Royal Society of Medicine Press Ltd

Published by the Royal Society of Medicine Press Ltd
1 Wimpole Street, London W1G 0AE, UK
Tel: +44 (0)20 7290 2921
Fax: +44 (0)20 7290 2929
Email: publishing@rsm.ac.uk
Website: www.rsmpress.co.uk

British Library Cataloguing in Publication Data
A catalogue record for this book is available from the British Library

ISBN 1-85315-598-5
ISSN 0143 6953

Distribution in Europe and Rest of World:
Marston Book Services Ltd
PO Box 269
Abingdon
Oxon OX14 4YN, UK
Tel: +44 (0)1235 465500
Fax: +44 (0)1235 465555
Email: direct.order@marston.co.uk

Distribution in the USA and Canada:
Royal Society of Medicine Press Ltd
c/o Jamco Distribution Inc
1401 Lakeway Drive
Lewisville, TX 75057, USA
Tel: +1 800 538 1287
Fax: +1 972 353 1303
Email: jamco@majors.com

Distribution in Australia and New Zealand:
Elsevier Australia
30-52 Smidmore Street
Marrikville NSW 2204, Australia
Tel: +61 2 9517 8999
Fax: +61 2 9517 2249
Email: service@elsevier.com.au

Commissioning editor - Peter Richardson
Editorial assistant - Hannah Wessely

Editorial services and typesetting by GM & BA Haddock, Ford, Midlothian, UK
Printed in The Netherlands by Alfabase, Alphen aan den Rijn

Contents

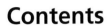

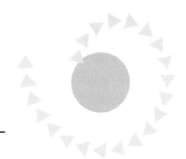

Contributors

Malcolm R. Alison DSc FRCPath
Professor, Centre for Diabetes and Metabolic Medicine, Institute of Cell and Molecular Science, Whitechapel, London and Histopathology Unit, Cancer Research UK, London, UK

Alastair D. Burt BSc MD FRCPath FIBiol
Dean of Clinical Medicine and Professor of Pathology, Department of Cellular Pathology, Royal Victoria Infirmary, and School of Clinical and Laboratory Sciences, University of Newcastle upon Tyne, Newcastle upon Tyne, UK

Simon S. Cross MD FRCPath
Reader, Academic Unit of Pathology, Division of Genomic Medicine, School of Medicine and Biomedical Sciences, University of Sheffield, Sheffield, UK

Natalie C. Direkze MA MB BS MRCP
Clinical Research Fellow, Histopathology Unit, Cancer Research UK, London, UK

Andrew R. Dodson MPhil CSci FIBMS
Diagnostic Development Quality Manager, Department of Cellular Pathology and Molecular Genetics, University of Liverpool, Liverpool, UK

Cyril Fisher MA MD DSc FRCPath
Professor of Tumour Pathology, Department of Histopathology, Royal Marsden Hospital, London, UK

Christopher S. Foster MD PhD DSc FASCP FRCPath
Professor of Cellular Pathology and Molecular Genetics, University of Liverpool, Liverpool, UK

Beate Haugk MD MRCPath
Consultant Histopathologist, Department of Cellular Pathology, Royal Victoria Infirmary, Newcastle upon Tyne, UK

Matthew J. Lovell MB BS BSc MRCP
Clinical Research Fellow, Histopathology Unit, Cancer Research UK, London, UK

Richard Poulsom PhD DSc FRCPath
Professor, Histopathology Unit, Cancer Research UK, London, UK

Jeffrey S. Ross MD
Cyrus Strong Merrill Professor and Chair, Department of Pathology and
Laboratory Medicine, Albany Medical College, Albany, New York, USA and
Division of Oncology Molecular Medicine, Millennium Pharmaceuticals, Inc.,
Cambridge, Massachusetts, USA

Roger D. Start MD FRCPath
Consultant Histpathologist, Department of Histopathology, Chesterfield
Royal Hospital, Calow, Derbyshire, UK

Timothy J. Stephenson MA MD MBA FRCPath
Consultant Histopathologist, Department of Histopathology, Royal
Hallamshire Hospital, Sheffield Teaching Hospitals NHS Trust, Sheffield, UK

Kevin P. West BSc MB ChB DMJ FRCPath
Consultant Histopathologist, University Hospitals of Leicester NHS Trust,
Leicester Royal Infirmary, Leicester, UK

Beate Haugk Alastair D. Burt

1

Non-alcoholic fatty liver disease

Non-alcoholic steatohepatitis (NASH), a liver disease histologically similar to alcoholic hepatitis but occurring in the absence of alcohol abuse, is an increasingly recognised and important cause of morbidity and mortality, particularly in the industrialised world. NASH was first described by Ludwig *et al.* in 1980[1] as 'a poorly understood and hitherto unnamed liver disease'. Since then, NASH has been subject of intensive investigation; we now recognise 'primary' non-alcoholic steatohepatitis as a stage within the spectrum of non-alcoholic fatty liver disease (NAFLD). NAFLD is becoming the preferred term and its spectrum ranges from simple steatosis through steatohepatitis, steatosis with fibrosis to cirrhosis.[2] Non-alcoholic fatty liver disease represents the hepatic manifestation of the metabolic syndrome which is defined as the presence of three of the following five components: (i) central obesity; (ii) hyperglycaemia (type 2 diabetes); (iii) low levels of high-density lipoprotein cholesterol; (iv) hypertriglyceridaemia; and (v) hypertension.[3] It should be differentiated from steatosis and steatohepatitis due to 'secondary', non-alcoholic causes such as drugs, toxins, genetic and metabolic diseases, malnutrition and gastrojejunal bypass surgery (Table 1).[2]

EPIDEMIOLOGY

Assessment of the prevalence of NAFLD is difficult. First, there are no specific serological markers for the diagnosis of NAFLD; liver enzyme tests may be entirely normal. Second, the disease can present in a variety of clinical settings:

Beate Haugk MD MRCPath
Consultant Histopathologist, Department of Cellular Pathology, Royal Victoria Infirmary, Newcastle upon Tyne NE1 4LP, UK

Alastair D. Burt BSc MD FRCPath FIBiol (for correspondence)
Dean of Clinical Medicine and Professor of Pathology, Department of Cellular Pathology, Royal Victoria Infirmary, Newcastle upon Tyne NE1 4LP, and School of Clinical and Laboratory Sciences, University of Newcastle upon Tyne, Newcastle upon Tyne NE2 4HH, UK (E-mail: a.d.burt@ncl.ac.uk)

Table 1 Causes of secondary non-alcoholic steatohepatitis (*modified from* Chitturi and Farrell[9])

Nutritional
    Total parenteral nutrition
    Jejunal diverticulosis
    Fasting/starvation
    Protein-calorie malnutrition

Drugs
  Cardiovascular
    Amiodarone
    Perhexiline maleate
    Coralgil (4′4′-diethylaminoethoxyhexoestrol)
    Nifedipine, diltiazem (calcium channel blockers)
  Hormones and hormone receptor ligands
    Glucocorticoids
    Synthetic oestrogens
    Tamoxifen
  Others
    Methotrexate
    Chloroquine
    Hycanthone

Surgical procedures
    Gastroplasty
    Jejuno-ileal bypass
    Jejunocolic bypass
    Biliopancreatic diversion
    Massive small intestinal resection

Metabolic and genetic disorders
    αβ-lipoproteinaemia
    Weber-Christian disease
    Type 1 glycogen storage disease
    Lipodystrophy
    Insulin receptor mutations

Environmental toxins
    Dimethylformamide
    Toxic oil syndrome (adulterated rapeseed cooking oil)

Others
    Inflammatory bowel disease

patients are often obese and/or diabetic, but they may also be lean and non-diabetic and, furthermore, the disease may be clinically silent. Third, a significant number of cases of cryptogenic cirrhosis may represent end-stage NAFLD leading to an underestimate of the overall number of cases. Fourth, the accurate diagnosis of NAFLD in any given setting still requires a liver biopsy – an invasive test. Furthermore, the definition of insignificant alcohol use in published studies is variable ranging from < 20 g/week to < 140 g/week.[3]

Investigations leading to a diagnosis of NAFLD are often triggered by the presence of elevated serum transaminases. Fatty liver, confirmed by histology, is present in 30–40% of patients with slightly elevated liver enzymes in the absence of alcohol abuse, viral hepatitis, autoimmune liver disease or congenital liver disease. A further 15–30% show steatohepatitis with varying degrees of fibrosis.[4] However, the prevalence of NAFLD may have been underestimated as cases with normal liver enzymes were not recognised. Recently, clinical data and serological results from more than 15,000 subjects for the third U.S. National Health and Nutrition Examination Survey (1988–1994; NHANES III) were analysed.[5,6] From this, one group estimated the prevalence of NAFLD in the US population to be 2.8% using elevated alanine aminotransferase (ALT) alone as a surrogate marker in the absence of any evidence of other liver disease. A fasting level of > 43 U/l was used as defined in the NHANES III manuals. If recently suggested lower levels of ALT (> 30 U/l for men and > 19 U/l for women) had been used, the prevalence would have risen to 12.4% for men and 13.9% for women.[5,7] In a separate analysis, Clark et al.[6] included abnormal aspartate aminotransferase (AST; > 37 U/l for men and > 31 U/l for women) and using the same lower values for ALT estimated 21.2% of the study population with unexplained elevated liver enzyme values to have NAFLD. Both studies, however, presumed these cases to be NAFLD without histological proof. Such analyses highlight the problems in the epidemiological study of a disease in which the gold standard diagnostic test remains the assessment of a liver biopsy – an invasive test required not only to prove NAFLD in the presence of otherwise unexplained liver enzyme elevations but also to exclude marker-negative liver diseases of different origin.[3,7] Despite the highlighted difficulties, there is no question that NAFLD affects a significant proportion of the general population world-wide. The prevalence in various populations probably ranges between 10–40%.[2,8] The prevalence of NASH within NAFLD ranges from 2% to 30%.[3,8]

PATHOGENESIS

There is a strong association between NAFLD and obesity, type 2 diabetes and hyperlipidaemia. One of the key pathogenetic factors for NAFLD appears to be insulin resistance which is strongly related to the metabolic syndrome and appears to be specific and an essential requirement for NASH independent of body weight.[9,10] Insulin resistance is defined as a smaller than expected response to a given dose of insulin. Insulin stimulates the deposition of glycogen and fat and the synthesis of proteins while inhibiting their breakdown. The liver manifests all the anabolic actions of insulin. It is the primary target and also the major processor for insulin: half of the secreted insulin never reaches the systemic circulation. In insulin resistance, there is an increase in circulating free fatty acids due to an attenuated inhibition of lipolysis by insulin leading to the accumulation of visceral fat.[11]

The pathogenetic mechanisms leading to insulin resistance are not fully understood. Recently, it has been found that inhibitor kinase kappa beta (IKκ-β), which interacts with nuclear factor kappa beta, is chronically elevated in insulin resistance. It has been shown that insulin resistance can be abolished by inhibiting IKκ-β. The mechanisms leading to sustained IKκ-β activation are still under investigation. TNF-α, a recognised activator of IKκ-β,[3,4] is a fat-derived peptide with a demonstrated inhibitory effect on insulin action by down-regulating the insulin-induced phosphorylation of insulin receptor substrate (IRS)-1.[2,12] Studies also suggest that dysregulated intramuscular fatty acid metabolism and excess lipid (lipotoxicity) have an important causative role in insulin resistance.[13] Fatty acids may cause insulin resistance by activation of a serine kinase cascade, leading to decreased insulin-stimulated insulin receptor substrate (IRS)-1 tyrosine phosphorylation and decreased IRS-1-associated phosphatidylinositol-3-kinase activity, an essential step in insulin-stimulated glucose transport into muscle.[14] Other molecules have been suggested as pathogenetic mediators for insulin resistance: PC-1, a cell surface glycoprotein; Rad, a member of the GTPase superfamily; and leptin, which induces dephosphorylation of IRS-1.[2]

Insulin resistance causes hepatic steatosis by favouring peripheral lipolysis with increased hepatic uptake of fatty acids and by hyperinsulinaemia. Insulin resistance also causes excess glycolysis with an increase in *de-novo* synthesis of free fatty acids. Disturbances of the fatty acid oxidation systems also play an important role. In the liver, fatty acids are oxidised in three organelles – the mitochondria, the peroxisomes and the microsomes. Mitochondrial β-oxidation converts free fatty acids to acetyl-CoA which can subsequently generate ATP (the major source of energy for the cell) via the respiratory chain. With insulin resistance, the accompanying hyperinsulinaemia has a direct effect on mitochondrial β-oxidation by inhibiting the transport of long-chain fatty acids from the cytosol into the mitochondria.[9] Hyperinsulinaemia also affects the complex mechanism of triglyceride assembly and export via degradation of apoprotein B,[3,15] further increasing the fat content within hepatocytes.

While these metabolic changes explain the accumulation of fat in hepatocytes, they do not account for all features of NASH. It has been postulated that a second hit is required for the development of an inflammatory lesion.[16] Oxidative stress is considered the main mechanism for the progression from steatosis to steatohepatitis. Oxidative stress results from an imbalance of pro-oxidants and antioxidants. Under physiological conditions, mitochondria are the main source of reactive oxygen species. Increased influx of free fatty acids may initially lead to an increase in β-oxidation leading to an increase in reactive oxygen species. This may lead to up-regulation of uncoupling protein 2 (UCP2) as a defence mechanism against reactive oxygen species but at the cost of ATP recovery.[17] The impairment of mitochondrial β-oxidation in established insulin resistance leads to induction of microsomal and peroxisomal oxidation systems. In particular, induction of microsomal cytochrome CYP2E1 and CYP4A have been implicated as a source of reactive oxygen species. A further potential pro-oxidant includes hydrogen peroxide derived from the peroxisomal oxidation system.[9] The genes encoding peroxisomal, microsomal and certain mitochondrial fatty acid metabolising enzymes in the liver are transcriptionally regulated by peroxisome proliferator-activated receptor alpha (PPAR-α) which up-regulates UCP2 and may also play a role in the pathogenesis of NASH.[18] In addition, there appears to be depletion of reduced glutathione (GSH) due to a defect in its uptake into the mitochondria leading to a decrease in antioxidants.[9]

Reactive oxygen species may lead to: (i) lipid peroxidation; (ii) cytokine production; and (iii) Fas ligand expression. Lipid peroxidation products alter mitochondrial DNA and also inhibit electron transfer along the respiratory chain. Reactive oxygen species mediate the release of TNF-α by hepatocytes, Kupffer cells and adipose tissue. Furthermore, the lipid peroxidation product 4-hydroxynonenal up-regulates transforming growth factor beta (TGF-β)

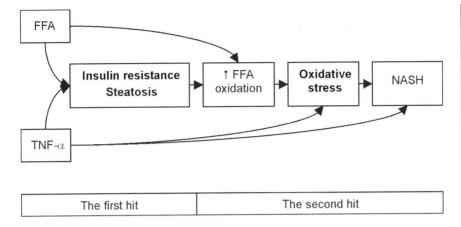

| The first hit | The second hit |

Fig. 1 Principal pathogenetic mechanism leading to NASH.

expression in macrophages. Interleukin 8 (IL-8), a potent chemo-attractant for neutrophils, is a further cytokine which may be released due to oxidative stress. Finally, reactive oxygen species can cause Fas ligand expression leading to hepatocyte death.[9] The above mentioned ATP depletion due to induction of UCP2 may worsen any injury.

This model of NASH pathogenesis, in which increased free fatty acids together with TNF-α lead to steatosis and insulin resistance (first hit) and then via oxidative stress (second hit) to steatohepatitis (Fig. 1), could explain all the typical morphological features of NASH.[19] For example, cytokines attract neutrophils, while hepatocyte death may be mediated by Fas ligand expression, mitochondrial permeability changes and cytokines. 4-Hydroxy-nonenal and malondialdehyde will cause cross linkage of proteins explaining Mallory bodies.[20] Metabolic zonation, reflecting the gradient of oxygen tension in the liver, accounts for the distribution of changes, particularly in the perivenular zones.[11] Fibrosis, which is clinically the most critical aspect of NASH as chronic liver disease, may be due to the activation of stellate cells by inflammatory mediators. Hyperinsulinaemia, hyperglycaemia and leptin have also been considered as profibrogenic.[3]

While this is a plausible model, it does not explain the variation in susceptibility for developing NASH rather than simple steatosis. Multiple host genetic factors and polymorphisms probably influence the individual risk of NASH.[3] Candidate genes include those which influence severity of steatosis, fatty acid oxidation, magnitude of oxidative stress, TNF-α expression and immunological effects.[21]

HISTOPATHOLOGY

STEATOSIS

Steatosis as part of NAFLD is usually macrovesicular in type and, akin to steatosis associated with alcohol excess, often perivenular in distribution. Up to 5% of steatosis can probably be regarded as within normal limits.[3,22] Simple steatosis is usually not accompanied by any significant inflammation but lipogranulomas can be seen due to rupture of lipid vacuoles. These can sometimes be difficult to distinguish from other granulomas or focal inflammation and the characteristic feature is that of epithelioid macrophages surrounding a central lipid droplet; eosinophils, lymphocytes and giant cells can also be seen.[22]

STEATOHEPATITIS

The 'classical' features of steatohepatitis include steatosis with liver cell ballooning, intracytoplasmic Mallory bodies, inflammatory infiltrates (predominantly neutrophils) and both perivenular and pericellular (chicken-wire) fibrosis.[23] These features are common to alcoholic and non-alcoholic steatohepatitis. It is now accepted, however, that not all features need to be present to make a diagnosis of steatohepatitis. The essential features for a diagnosis of steatohepatitis and its demarcation from simple steatosis are not yet unequivocally defined. Scheuer and Lefkowitch[23] described the essential components of alcoholic hepatitis as liver-cell damage, inflammation and fibrosis with fatty change usually but not invariably present. Fibrosis is probably a constant feature and, if not present, the diagnosis of alcoholic hepatitis should be at least questioned.[22,23] A survey of international hepatopathologists (all of whom have published on NAFLD and NASH) suggested that even steatosis was not accepted by all as an essential feature for the diagnosis of NASH. Some emphasised the greater importance of cell injury such as ballooning. Ballooning was a required feature for 60% of the group; the remaining surveyed pathologists regarded it as one of three features to be considered in the diagnostic criteria of which at least two should be present. Lobular inflammation was an essential feature for only half of pathologists surveyed. With regards to the components of the inflammatory infiltrate, a minority regarded neutrophils as a requirement and the remainder regarded them as either common or helpful. Whether fibrosis is a necessary feature for NASH is also under discussion. Of surveyed pathologists, 20% required perisinusoidal fibrosis whereas 80% found it common but not essential. Portal fibrosis in the absence of perisinusoidal fibrosis was considered unusual (80%) in adult NASH. Mallory bodies do not seem to be a requirement for NASH and, by definition, absence of Mallory bodies does not militate against the diagnosis of NASH.[3]

In the light of these difficulties, can we actually diagnose NASH? It is important to recognise the overall pattern of injury; features must never be assessed out of context. Lesions in NASH commonly show a zone-3 predominance (perivenular distribution). Hepatopathologists agree that adult NASH is characterised by a combination of features in which steatosis, ballooning, lobular inflammation and perisinusoidal fibrosis are the main lesions of interest.[3] As noted above, none of these four components is felt to be an absolute requirement, but the majority of hepatopathologists would rely on three of these four components for the diagnosis. Furthermore, the fewer features are observed, the more prominent these should be to ensure a confident diagnosis. Steatosis, ballooning and inflammation may indicate a recent or persisting insult, and fibrosis is a reflection of an insult of some

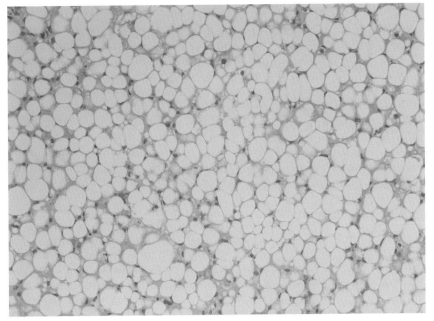

Fig. 2 Macrovesicular steatosis.

duration. The degree of injury and its resolution may depend on the metabolic status of the individual at the time of the biopsy.[3]

Steatosis

Steatosis is characterised by intracytoplasmic lipid droplets which in paraffin-processed, routinely stained sections will be represented by cytoplasmic

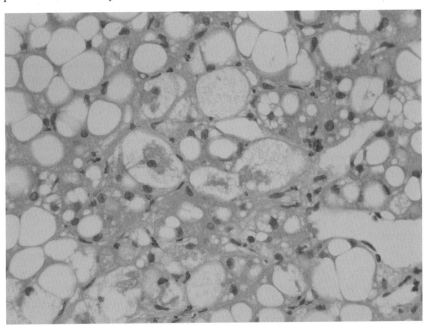

Fig. 3 Ballooning degeneration with Mallory body.

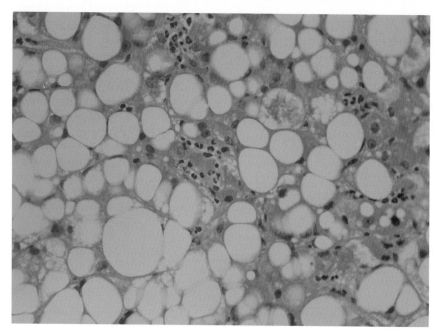

Fig. 4 Neutrophils surrounding a hepatocyte (satellitosis).

vacuoles. In NAFLD this is mainly macrovesicular in type, characterised by a single droplet displacing the nucleus to one side (Fig. 2). Microvesicular steatosis as a minor component can also be seen in which small droplets are dispersed in the cytoplasm without displacing the nucleus.[22]

Ballooning

As noted above, ballooning appears to be a very important component of steatohepatitis and it is critical to recognise this lesion. Ballooning degeneration is significant swelling of a hepatocyte with loss of the polygonal shape, a more central nucleus and abundant pale cytoplasm in the form of little strands. It is thought to be the structural manifestation of microtubular disruption and impaired protein secretion accompanied by fluid retention (Fig. 3).[22]

Lobular inflammation

Lobular inflammation is integral to the diagnosis of NASH but it is often mild. Lobular inflammation was seen in over 90% of published case series.[24] The inflammatory infiltrate is often mixed with a scattering of neutrophil polymorphs (Fig. 4). In our experience, neutrophil polymorphs are not always seen and their absence does not mitigate against the diagnosis of NASH.

Fibrosis

We feel that pericellular fibrosis is very important; it is interesting to note that pericellular fibrosis is regarded as a constant feature of alcoholic steatohepatitis[22,23] but it is given less emphasis in NASH. Fibrosis is mainly seen in zone 3 in a perisinusoidal and pericellular distribution (Fig. 5) but can also be seen in periportal areas, particularly in NASH in children. Fibrosis indicates a significant insult to the liver parenchyma and is, therefore, more

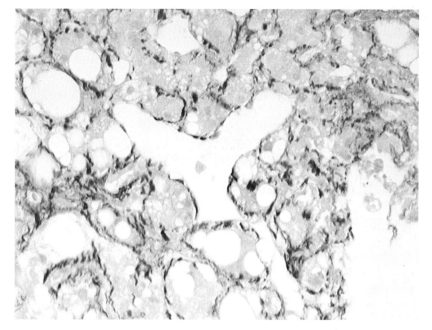

Fig. 5 Pericellular fibrosis in a perivenular distribution.

likely to indicate a progressive disease. It is not unusual to see 'steatosis with fibrosis' in the absence of significant inflammation or ballooning; this is recognised to be part of the spectrum of fatty liver disease.

Mallory bodies

Mallory bodies, when present, are quite often seen within ballooned hepatocytes and the presence of Mallory bodies is, without question, useful in supporting the diagnosis of steatohepatitis. Mallory bodies or Mallory's hyalin are perinuclear cytoplasmic clumps and strands of eosinophilic material composed of intermediate filaments of the cytoskeleton (Fig. 6). Mallory bodies are often poorly formed in NASH. The presence of Mallory bodies can be confirmed by immunohistochemistry using CK8, CK18, ubiquitin and p62.[3,22]

Other features

Nuclear glycogenation, mild portal inflammation, megamitochondria, apoptotic hepatocytes and iron deposition can also be seen in NASH. Most patients with NAFLD do not have significant iron accumulation and it does not seem to be associated with poorer clinical outcome.[25] Severe portal inflammation and interface hepatitis are not usually seen in steatohepatitis; they raise the possibility of a concomitant disease such as viral hepatitis (see below).

A frequently asked question is: can we distinguish NASH from alcoholic steatohepatitis (ASH)? There are features which have not been described in NASH but are seen in ASH including sclerosing hyalin necrosis, veno-occlusive lesions, ductular reaction and cholangiolitis and bilirubinostasis.[3,26] The latter three may reflect concomitant pancreatitis in alcoholic patients and

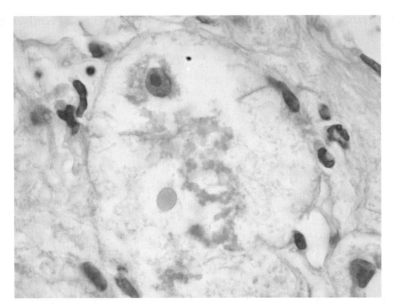

Fig. 6 Mallory body and giant mitochondrion in a ballooned hepatocyte.

are probably not a primary feature of the injury to the hepatocytes. Sclerosing hyalin necrosis describes confluent or central–central bridging necrosis which occasionally occurs in alcoholic hepatitis. Abundant Mallory bodies are regarded as strongly suggestive of ASH.[22,27] Mega or giant mitochondria can be seen in both NASH and ASH. Overall, nuclear glycogenation or clearing is much more common in NASH compared with ASH,[3] but it is not a specific feature nor a lesion associated with more progressive disease. Although NASH and ASH are histologically not identical, they share many features; in the great majority of cases, one would not be able to reliably distinguish them on histological grounds alone. Histopathologists should be cautious in labelling steatohepatitis as alcoholic in the absence of a firm clinical history.

GRADING AND SEVERITY

Once a diagnosis of steatosis or steatohepatitis has been made, the severity should be assessed. Steatosis is usually graded as mild (< 33% hepatocytes/parenchyma), moderate (> 33–66% hepatocytes/parenchyma) and severe (> 66% hepatocytes/parenchyma). With regard to hepatitis in general, there has traditionally been a tendency to describe the severity as mild, moderate or severe with some rather arbitrary boundaries. A histological activity index (HAI) for the assessment of chronic hepatitis, particularly hepatitis B and C, is now widely used. There are a number of different systems following the original description by Knodell in 1981, including the Metavir system and the HAI modified by Ishak.[28] Grading systems for steatohepatitis have been proposed, in particular to assess the growing number of biopsies with NAFLD and NASH. The grading system proposed by Brunt[3] distinguishes mild, moderate and severe and defines criteria for three grades as well as scoring the individual components numerically (Table 2). Matteoni

Table 2 Grading and staging the histopathological lesions of NASH (adapted from Brunt[3])

	Mild (Grade 1)	Moderate (Grade 2)	Severe (Grade 3)
Steatosis	Predominantly macro-vesicular. Involves < 33% up to 66% of the lobules	Any degree and usually mixed macrovesicular and microvesicular	Typically > 66% (panacinar), commonly mixed steatosis
Ballooning	Occasionally observed, zone 3 hepatocytes	Obvious and present in zone 3	Predominantly zone 3, marked
Lobular inflammation	Scattered and mild acute (polymorphs) inflammation and occasional chronic inflammation (mononuclear cells)	Polymorphs may be noted associated with ballooned hepatocytes, pericellular fibrosis; mild chronic inflammation may be seen	Scattered acute and chronic inflammation; polymorphs may appear concentrated in zone 3 areas of ballooning and perisinusoidal fibrosis
Portal inflammation	None or mild	Mild to moderate	Mild or moderate

Steatosis:
    1   0–33%
    2   33–66%
    3   > 66%

Ballooning: zonal location noted and severity (mild or marked) recorded to estimates of number of hepatocytes involved

Lobular inflammation: 0–3 based on observations of foci per x20 field, cell types (acute or chronic noted)
    1   1–2 foci
    2   up to 4 foci
    3   > 4 foci

Portal inflammation:
    1   Mild
    2   Moderate
    3   Severe

Staging fibrosis in NASH:
    Stage 1   Zone 3 perivenular perisinusoidal/pericellular fibrosis, focal or extensive
    Stage 2   As above with focal or extensive periportal fibrosis
    Stage 3   Bridging fibrosis, focal or extensive
    Stage 4   Cirrhosis

et al.[29] distinguished four histologically defined categories of fatty liver disease for prognostic purposes: group 1, fatty liver only; group 2, fat accumulation and non-specific inflammation; group 3, fat accumulation and ballooning degeneration; and group 4, fat accumulation, ballooning degeneration and either Mallory's hyalin or fibrosis. Steatonecrosis (ballooning degeneration) was associated with a higher incidence of cirrhosis and a higher liver disease-related mortality rate. This system only considers the presence or absence of

Table 3 NAFLD Activity Score (NAS) (*Adapted from* Kleiner et al.[30])

NECRO-INFLAMMATION			
Steatosis		0	< 5%
		1	0–33%
		2	33–66%
		3	> 66%
Ballooning		0	None
		1	Few
		2	Many/prominent
Lobular inflammation		0	None
		1	< 2 foci/200x
		2	2–4 foci/200x
		3	> 4 foci/200x
FIBROSIS			
Stage	0	None	
Stage	1a	Zone 3 perisinusoidal fibrosis, requires trichrome to see	
	1b	Zone 3 perisinusoidal fibrosis, no trichrome needed	
	1c	Fibrosis limited to portal tracts	
Stage	2	Stage 1a/b with periportal fibrosis	
Stage	3	Bridging fibrosis	
Stage	4	Cirrhosis	

ballooning degeneration without indication of how many hepatocytes are affected. Recently, a NAFLD Activity Score (NAS) has been proposed[30] which assesses steatosis, ballooning, lobular inflammation and fibrosis (Table 3). Kleiner and colleagues have suggested that this can derive an overall necro-inflammatory score from 0 to 8. The fibrosis is staged separately.

Currently, these scoring systems are used mainly for epidemiological studies and clinical trials. The criteria for mild, moderate or severe steatohepatitis cannot be defined numerically on the basis of available scoring systems until a large cohort of patients has been examined and the value of the individual lesions of steatohepatitis correlated with morbidity and mortality. However, the NAS appears to be a potentially valuable tool in the systematic assessment of NAFLD in liver biopsies. Its components may be scored individually and their severity described in the report. In addition to assessing the features of the NAS, a report may want to include comments on the presence or absence of Mallory's hyalin, lipogranulomas, megamitochondria, glycogenated nuclei, iron content and acidophil bodies. The severity of the portal inflammation may be assessed as mild, moderate or severe.

TERMINOLOGY

The term non-alcoholic steatohepatitis was coined in 1980 by Ludwig[1] and is now well established among pathologists and clinicians. Non-alcoholic fatty liver disease (NAFLD) was introduced to cover the entire spectrum of fatty liver disease which is not related to alcohol. However, the definition of a disease as 'NON-another disease' has been questioned by pathologists and clinicians and other names have been proposed. The use of MESH (MEtabolic syndrome SteatoHepatitis) or MSSH (Metabolic Syndrome SteatoHepatitis) in recognition of the association with the metabolic syndrome has been suggested.[3] In cases with a known association with drugs, DISH (Drug Induced SteatoHepatitis) has been proposed.[3] In agreement with Brunt,[3] we feel that as histopathologists we should not get entangled in any MSSH/MESH or 'DISH' out any diagnoses with an aetiological label but clearly state the pathological process, which will be either steatosis or steatohepatitis, and correlate it with the clinical history.

FURTHER CONSIDERATIONS

NATURAL HISTORY

The natural history of NAFLD is not well defined. It is clear that some patients with steatosis follow a progressive clinical course whereas others remain stable. It appears that 50% of cases with steatosis do not show any significant change on histology on follow-up biopsies, whereas 27% show fibrosis and 19% cirrhosis.[8] Few clinical data can distinguish those with a benign course from those with a progressive outcome. It has been suggested that age above 45 years, obesity, diabetes and an AST/ALT ratio > 1 are associated with an increased risk for fibrosis. These are criteria which may guide clinicians towards undertaking a liver biopsy.[8] Histologically proven ballooning degeneration of hepatocytes with fibrosis and Mallory's hyalin appears to indicate the aggressive form of NAFLD.[29]

NAFLD AND CRYPTOGENIC CIRRHOSIS

Cirrhosis is regarded as cryptogenic after exclusion of recognisable aetiologies. Possible underlying aetiologies include occult alcohol excess, occult viral (non-B, non-C) hepatitis, silent autoimmune hepatitis or progression of NASH.[31] It is now increasingly common to attribute cryptogenic cirrhosis to 'burnt out' NASH. Caldwell et al.[31] showed a prevalence of diabetes and obesity of over 70% among patients with cryptogenic cirrhosis suggesting that NASH plays an under-recognised role in many patients with cryptogenic cirrhosis. However, if 'end-stage' cirrhosis develops following biopsy-proven NASH, by definition this would not be cryptogenic cirrhosis. Hui et al.[32] proposed pathological criteria for the definition of NASH-related cirrhosis. The presence of steatosis and mixed inflammation would be regarded as definite, steatosis with only chronic inflammation as probable, steatosis or mixed inflammation only as possible and absence of steatosis and inflammation as cryptogenic.

NAFLD AND TRANSPLANTATION

The recurrence of NAFLD in transplanted livers is documented.[33,34] Kim et al.[34] describe six out of eight patients transplanted for NASH to develop persistent fatty infiltration. Three of these developed hepatocellular degeneration consistent with NASH.

PAEDIATRIC NAFLD

There is a rising incidence of NAFLD and NASH in children. Based on abnormal liver function tests and the prevalence of obesity it appears that > 1–2% of all American adolescents may have NAFLD.[35] Often, children are referred for different reasons when NAFLD is discovered. Clinically, they often present with obesity, hepatomegaly and acanthosis nigricans. Histologically, they show more severe steatosis and less ballooning, Mallory's hyalin and lobular inflammation compared with adulthood NASH. There is very little infiltration by neutrophils. By contrast, there is more portal-based inflammation and, strikingly, usually more portal fibrosis without perisinusoidal fibrosis; there is also an apparent lack of zone 3 predominance.[3,35]

NAFLD AND HEPATOCELLULAR CARCINOMA

The presence of HCC in NAFLD is documented.[27,36] One study[36] reported a 47% incidence of HCC in biopsy-proven NASH-related cirrhosis whereas in a separate study the incidence was zero.[32] Both studies were, however, looking at very small numbers. The incidence of HCC in cryptogenic cirrhosis may be similar to that in hepatitis C associated cirrhosis.[37]

CO-EXISTENCE OF NAFLD AND OTHER LIVER DISEASES

In a retrospective study in St Louis, it was shown that steatohepatitis co-exists with other liver diseases in up to 5% of liver biopsies. In absolute numbers, steatohepatitis appears to co-exist most often with hepatitis C. Although steatosis is observed in hepatitis C, in particular in genotype 3, co-existence of hepatitis C and steatohepatitis appears to be an overlap of two common diseases.[38]

SECONDARY NASH

Primary NASH refers to conditions which are related to insulin resistance. There are a number of different non-alcoholic causes for steatosis and steatohepatitis with different pathogeneses and clinical outcomes which are often described as secondary NAFLD or NASH 2 (Table 1). Causes for secondary NAFLD/NASH include drugs, in particular amiodarone and perhexiline maleate, which cause steatohepatitis through mitochondrial injury.[9] Corticosteroids, tamoxifen and oestrogens exacerbate insulin resistance, diabetes and hypertriglyceridaemia.[39] Jejuno-ileal bypass surgery for the treatment of obesity is another well-described cause of secondary NASH, although the procedure has now been largely abandoned. Steatohepatitis is thought to have been caused by a combination of pre-existing steatosis/steatohepatitis, micronutrient deficiency and bacterial overgrowth with associated endotoxin injury. Profound weight loss and starvation can also cause secondary NASH via induction of Cyp 2E1. Total parenteral nutrition has been reported to cause steatohepatitis due to carbohydrate overload and micronutrient deficiency.[9] Rarer causes include a-β/hypo-β-lipoproteinaemia, Weber-Christian disease and some environmental toxins.[40]

THERAPEUTIC STRATEGIES

The first-line therapeutic approach to NAFLD is the treatment of the associated conditions. Weight reduction, particularly in NAFLD related to obesity, appears the obvious measure and many studies have shown a significant biochemical and histological improvement of NAFLD following weight loss. However, in some, particularly in cases where there was rapid weight loss and starvation, necro-inflammation and fibrosis developed. Both the rate and degree of weight loss appear to be important; gradual weight loss appears to lead to improvement.[40] In type 2 diabetes, good management of the hyperglycaemia will improve NAFLD.

In total parenteral nutrition and jejuno-ileal bypass surgery associated (secondary) NASH treatment with choline and antibiotics led to improvement.[40] Withdrawal of drugs and toxins causing steatohepatitis will also lead to resolution.

Drug treatments for NAFLD include the lipid-lowering drug gemfibrozil, the cell membrane stabilising ursodeoxycholic acid and betaine, which reduces deposition of triglyceride. N-Acetyl cysteine increases glutathione levels and vitamin E is an antioxidant. Further drugs specifically target insulin resistance. Metformin appears to inhibit the expression of TNF-α and thiazolidinediones selectively enhance or partially mimic certain actions of insulin. Rosiglitazone is such an agent which led to a significant improvement.[40] There have not been, as yet, any large randomised clinical trials for any of these agents. It is likely that, over the next 5 years, a clearer picture will emerge for therapeutic intervention in NAFLD/NASH. Histological assessment of severity of disease will then become even more important in managing such patients.

Points for best practice

- 'Primary' non-alcoholic steatohepatitis (NASH) is part of the spectrum of non-alcoholic fatty liver disease (NAFLD) which includes steatosis, steatohepatitis and cirrhosis. NAFLD has become the preferred term.

- NAFLD is the hepatic manifestation of the metabolic syndrome. 'Secondary' NASH is due to a variety of causes including drugs, metabolic, nutritional and genetic disorders, toxins and surgical procedures.

- The main histological components of NASH are steatosis, ballooning degeneration, lobular inflammation and pericellular fibrosis. Most hepatopathologists would rely on three out of these four components for the diagnosis of NASH.

- The presence of Mallory's hyalin is helpful in supporting a diagnosis of NASH but its absence does not mitigate against a diagnosis of NASH.

- Alcoholic steatohepatitis and non-alcoholic steatohepatitis are not identical. However, they share many features and it is often not possible to distinguish them on histological grounds alone.

Points for best practice *(continued)*

- Pathologists should exert great caution in labelling steatohepatitis as being of a particular aetiology on the basis of morphology. A histopathological diagnosis of steatosis, steatohepatitis or cirrhosis should be made and subsequently correlated with the clinical history.

- Paediatric NASH more often shows portal based fibrosis and inflammation together with severe steatosis. It often shows less ballooning degeneration, lobular inflammation and pericellular fibrosis.

- Grading and staging of NAFLD is mainly performed in the context of epidemiological studies and clinical trials. The NAFLD Activity Index (NAS) is a potentially valuable tool in the systematic assessment of NAFLD in liver biopsies and its components could be scored and described in the report.

References

1. Ludwig J, Viggiano TR, McGill DB, Beverly JO. Non-alcoholic steatohepatitis: Mayo Clinic experiences with a hitherto unnamed disease. *Mayo Clin Proc* 1980; **55**: 434–438.
2. Angulo P. Non-alcoholic fatty liver disease. *N Engl J Med* 2002; **346**: 1221–1231.
3. Brunt EM. Non-alcoholic steatohepatitis. *Semin Liver Dis* 2004; **24**: 3–20.
4. Clark JM, Brancati FL, Diehl AM. Non-alcoholic liver disease. *Gastroenterology* 2002; **122**: 1649–1657.
5. Ruhl CE, Everhart JE. Determinants of the association of overweight with elevated serum alanine aminotransferase activity in the United States. *Gastroenterology* 2003; **124**: 71–79.
6. Clark JM, Brancati FL, Diehl AM. The prevalence and etiology of elevated aminotransferase levels in the United States. *Am J Gastroenterol* 2003; **98**: 960–967.
7. Clark JM, Diehl AM. Defining non-alcoholic fatty liver disease: implications for epidemiologic studies. *Gastroenterology* 2003; **124**: 248–250.
8. Falck-Ytter Y, Younossi ZM, Marchesini G, McCullough AJ. Clinical features and natural history of non-alcoholic steatosis syndromes. *Semin Liver Dis* 2001; **21**: 17–26.
9. Chitturi S, Farrell GC. Etiopathogenesis of non-alcoholic steatohepatitis. *Semin Liver Dis* 2001; **21**: 27–41.
10. Chitturi S, Abeygunasekera S, Farrell GC *et al*. NASH and insulin resistance: insulin hypersecretion and specific association with the insulin resistance syndrome. *Hepatology* 2002; **35**: 373–379.
11. Browning JD, Horton JD. Molecular mediators of hepatic steatosis and liver injury. *J Clin Invest* 2004; **11**: 147–152.
12. Hotamisligil GS. Inflammatory pathways and insulin action. *Int J Obes Relat Metab Disord* 2003; **27 (Suppl 3)**: 53–55.
13. Peterson KF, Dufour S, Befroy D, Garcia R, Shulman G. Impaired mitochondrial activity in the insulin-resistant offspring of patients with type 2 diabetes. *N Engl J Med* 2004; **350**: 664–671.
14. Petersen KF, Shulman GI. Pathogenesis of skeletal muscle insulin resistance in type 2 diabetes mellitus. *Am J Cardiol* 2002; **90(5A)**: 11G–18G.
15. Charlton M, Sreekumar R, Rasmussen D, Lindor K, Nair KS. Apolipoprotein synthesis in non-alcoholic steatohepatitis. *Hepatology* 2002; **35**: 898–904.
16. Day CP, James OFW. Steatohepatitis: a tale of two 'hits'? *Gastroenterology* 1998; **114**: 842–845.

17. Chavin KD, Yang S, Lin HZ *et al.* Obesity induces expression of uncoupling protein-2 in hepatocytes and promotes liver ATP depletion. *J Biol Chem* 1999; **274**: 5692–5700.
18. Rao MS, Reddy JK. Peroxisomal beta-oxidation and steatohepatitis. *Semin Liver Dis* 2001; **21**: 43–55.
19. James OFW, Day CP. Non-alcoholic steatohepatitis: another disease of affluence [Commentary]. *Lancet* 1999; **353**: 1634–1636.
20. Pessayre D, Berson A, Fromenty B, Mansouri A. Mitochondria in steatohepatitis. *Semin Liver Dis* 2001; **21**: 57–69.
21. Day CP. The potential role of genes in non-alcoholic fatty liver disease. *Clin Liver Dis* 2004; **8**: 673–691.
22. Burt AD, Mutton A, Day C. Diagnosis and interpretation of steatosis and steatohepatitis. *Semin Diagn Pathol* 1998; **15**: 246–258.
23. Scheuer PJ, Lefkowitch JH. *Liver Biopsy Interpretation*. London: W.B. Saunders, 1994.
24. Brunt EM. Non-alcoholic steatohepatitis: definition and pathology. *Semin Liver Dis* 2001; **21**: 3–16.
25. Younossi ZM, Gramlich T, Bacon BR *et al.* Hepatic iron and non-alcoholic fatty liver disease. *Hepatology* 1999; **30**: 847–850.
26. Brunt EM. Alcoholic and non-alcoholic steatohepatitis. *Clin Liver Dis* 2002; **6**: 399–420.
27. Ludwig J, Mcgill DB, Lindor KD. Review: non-alcoholic steatohepatitis. *J Gastroenterol Hepatol* 1997; **12**: 398–403.
28. Brunt EM. Grading and staging the histopathological lesions of chronic hepatitis: the Knodell histology activity index and beyond. *Hepatology* 2000; **31**: 241–246.
29. Matteoni CA, Younossi ZM, Gramlich T *et al.* Non-alcoholic fatty liver disease: a spectrum of clinical and pathological severity. *Gastroenterology* 1999; **116**: 1413–1419.
30. Kleiner DE, Brunt EM, Van Natta M *et al.* Design and validation of a histologic scoring system for non-alcoholic fatty liver disease (NAFLD) and non-alcoholic steatohepatitis (NASH). *Hepatology* 2003; **38**: 233A.
31. Caldwell SH, Oelsner DH, Iezzoni JC *et al.* Cryptogenic cirrhosis: clinical characterization and risk factors for underlying disease. *Hepatology* 1999; **29**: 664–669.
32. Hui JM, Kench JG, Chitturi S *et al.* Long-term outcomes of cirrhosis in non-alcoholic steatohepatitis compared with hepatitis C. *Hepatology* 2003; **38**: 420–427.
33. Molloy RM, Komorowski R, Varma RR. Recurrent non-alcoholic steatohepatitis and cirrhosis after liver transplantation. *Liver Transpl Surg* 1997; **3**: 177–178.
34. Kim WR, Poterucha JJ, Porayko MK *et al.* Recurrence of non-alcoholic steatohepatitis following liver transplantation. *Transplantation* 1996; **62**: 8102–8105.
35. Lavine JE, Schwimmer JB. Non-alcoholic fatty liver disease in the pediatric population. *Clin Liver Dis* 2004; **8**: 549–558.
36. Shimada M, Hashimoto E, Taniai M *et al.* Hepatocellular carcinoma in patients with non-alcoholic steatohepatitis. *J Hepatol* 2002; **37**: 154–160.
37. Ratziu V, Bonyhay L, Di Martino V *et al.* Survival, liver failure and hepatocellular carcinoma in obesity-related cryptogenic cirrhosis. *Hepatology* 2002; **35**: 1485–1493.
38. Brunt EM, Ramrakhiani S, Cordes BG *et al.* Concurrence of histologic features of steatohepatitis with other forms of chronic liver disease. *Modern Pathol* 2003; **16**: 49–56.
39. Farrell GC. Drugs and steatohepatitis. *Semin Liv Dis* 2002; **22**: 185–194.
40. Angulo P, Lindor KD. Treatment of non-alcoholic fatty liver: present and emerging therapies. *Semin Liver Dis* 2001; **21**: 81–88.

Kevin P. West

2

Histopathology training in the UK: present tense – future perfect?

Postgraduate medical education in the UK has undergone major changes over recent years and further reforms are under way. The changes have concerned both the structure and content of training. This article will review the changes, outline the arrangements currently being put into place and look at possible future developments, particularly with respect to the content of training curricula. For the purposes of this article, the term histopathology will be used to incorporate cytopathology, forensic pathology, paediatric pathology and neuropathology.

THE PAST

Until 1996 trainees spent:

- Approximately 1 year in senior house officer (SHO) posts (often rotating through different pathology disciplines).

- Approximately 2 years in the registrar grade during which time they were required to pass the Primary MRCPath examination.

- 2–3 years in the senior registrar grade culminating in successful completion of the Final MRCPath examination.

At this time, there was no specialist register. Possession of the MRCPath qualification was taken as evidence of suitability for a consultant appointment and there was little in the way of formal review of progress in training.

DRIVERS FOR CHANGE IN HISTOPATHOLOGY TRAINING

In 1996, following the Calman Report,[1] the registrar and senior registrar grades were merged to form the specialist registrar (SpR) grade. Thus, the competitive

Kevin P. West BSc MB ChB DMJ FRCPath
Consultant Histopathologist, University Hospitals of Leicester NHS Trust, Leicester Royal Infirmary, Leicester LE1 5WW, UK (E-mail: kpw2@leicester.ac.uk)

hurdle between the two previous grades was removed and higher specialist training became seamless. At the same time, and unrelated to the proposed reforms, there was a severe reduction in the number of trainees in histopathology. This reduction followed concerns that there were too many trainees relative to the number of consultant posts available. These fears eventually proved to be unfounded but they heralded the start of a severe workforce crisis that is not yet resolved.

In addition to developing the specialist registrar grade, the Calman Report recommended the introduction of an annual review of progress known as the Record of in Training Assessment (RITA) which is described in *A Guide to Specialist Registrar Training*.[2] The purpose of this was to provide a more rigorous assessment of trainees, allowing identification of problems at an early stage and informing appropriate corrective action.

The Royal College of Pathologists (RCPath) examination structure changed at about this time. The Part 1 examination replaced the Primary MRCPath and no longer involved an assessment in all disciplines of pathology. For this reason, many of the rotating SHO posts became discipline-specific offering training in one branch of pathology. These posts, although nominally for one year, were often extended to allow time for a trainee to secure a further post.

On appointment to the SpR grade, a date was calculated for the award of a Certificate of Completion of Specialist Training (CCST), the period of training being defined by the RCPath subject to approval by the Specialist Training Authority (STA) of the Medical Royal Colleges (<sta-mrc.org.uk> 2004). For histopathology, the time required in the SpR grade was 4.5 years and appointment to the grade was contingent upon having completed at least one year of SHO training. Thus, training became more strictly time limited. Previously, trainees could bide their time in a training post whilst waiting for a particular consultant vacancy. Although this was advantageous to trainees, the effect was to block training posts and reduce the throughput of the training system.

WORKFORCE PLANNING

In the late 1990s, a considerable gap appeared between the predicted output of training programmes and the number of consultant vacancies in histopathology. By 2000, it was acknowledged that urgent action was required in order to meet the demands of both consultant retirement and consultant expansion. By this time, many hospitals were short-staffed and some histopathology departments were left with no consultants.

One of the driving forces for consultant expansion was the *National Cancer Plan*,[3] which followed the Calman-Hine report.[4] These gave histopathology a pivotal role in cancer care through the establishment of multidisciplinary teams for each cancer site.

Following discussions between the RCPath and the Department of Health, a decision was made to increase the number of doctors entering training in histopathology in England by the creation of so-called SHO Schools.

SHO SCHOOLS

The histopathology SHO Schools initiative was funded through the National Cancer Plan. In 2001, eighteen SHOs were recruited – six each to Leeds, Leicester and Southampton. Recruitment was, for the first time ever, organised on a national basis and the recruits were of an exceptionally high calibre. In 2003, the intake for each of the three SHO Schools was increased to eight and plans were put in place for the development of a further nine schools. Three of these, Eastern, Newcastle and West Midlands, took their first groups of trainees in 2004 with the remainder planned for 2005.

Training in the SHO Schools is highly structured and the trainees come together for 4 weeks of block teaching during their 1-year posts. Whilst there is a considerable amount of group teaching, the apprenticeship model of histopathology training has, by no means, been abandoned.[5]

The SHO Schools developed a curriculum that has been incorporated into the RCPath histopathology curriculum, providing detailed objectives for trainees. A structured curriculum facilitated the refinement of the SHO Aptitude Assessment. Initially, this had largely been a paper exercise followed by a discussion of a portfolio of reports and a limited amount of microscopy with an external assessor. The SHO Schools developed the Aptitude Assessment for SHOs to incorporate an Objective Structured Pathology Examination (OSPE) in which competence may be assessed in a variety of contexts relevant to histopathology. In addition to the examination of macroscopic and microscopic images, the assessment may include stations covering topics such as consent and communication. This more structured approach will be used in the RCPath Year 1 Histopathology Assessment to be introduced in 2006 (see Fig. 1).

Training SHOs in groups offers some economy of scale when imparting basic knowledge. Learning with peers avoids the isolation felt by many single-handed SHOs. However, some disadvantages were also apparent.

In the past, many SHOs were able to secure SpR posts in the same department. Thus a degree of continuity was achieved. SHO Schools, on the other hand, were expected to export trainees after one year because there would be no possibility of offering six or eight SpR opportunities in any single training programme.

The contractual arrangements were also a potential source of difficulty as the posts were for a fixed 1-year period without the possibility for extension. Trainees could, therefore, have been left without a post at the end of the SHO year. This concern proved to be groundless as ample SpR opportunities were available.

Another potential problem arose as a result of funding for the SHO School posts. Many of the SHO posts in histopathology that existed prior to the establishment of the SHO Schools attracted additional duty payments for work extending beyond the standard 40-hour week. In most cases, the additional supplement was equivalent to 40% of the basic salary. Additional duty payments were not included in the funding for the new posts created for the SHO Schools as it was considered that training needs could be met within a 40-hour week. Concerns were expressed about the potential impact of the funding arrangements on recruitment but these have not been justified by events as there has been a large excess of applicants over available posts every year since the inception of the SHO Schools.

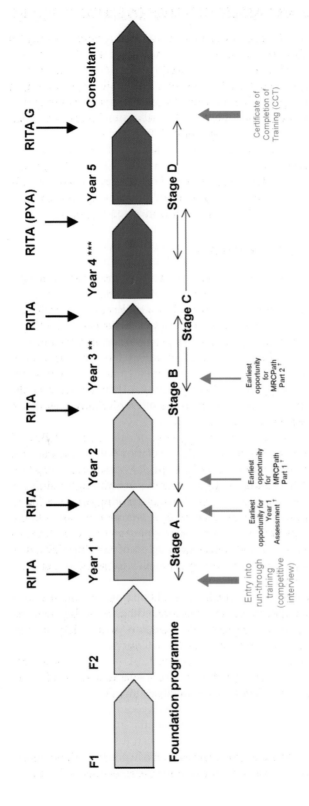

* Trainees must have passed the Year 1 Record of In-Training Assessment (RITA) by the end of Year 1.
  Failure to pass the Year 1 Assessment will prevent the trainee from progressing in the training grade.

** Trainees must have passed the Part 1 MRCPath examination by the end of Year 3.
   Failure to pass the Part 1 examination by the end of Year 3 will prevent the trainee from progressing to the next year of training.

*** Trainees must have passed the Part 2 MRCPath examination by the end of Year 4.
    Failure to pass the Part 2 examination by the end of Year 4 will prevent the trainee from progressing to the next year of training.

† Suggested earliest opportunity to attempt the Year 1 Assessment, Part 1 and Part 2 MRCPath examinations.

‡ Specialist training – either general histopathology, general surgical pathology or subspecialty training in cytopathology and dermatopathology, forensic pathology, neuropathology and paediatric pathology.

Fig. 1 Proposed histopathology run-through training model.

INTENSIVE TRAINING AND ASSESSMENT FOR OVERSEAS DOCTORS

There are substantial numbers of doctors with some previous training in histopathology who wish to complete their training in the UK. For the majority, it was considered that the appropriate route of entry to further training would be through SHO posts. However, for some, it was thought possible to effect a more rapid induction into UK histopathology training. For these candidates the concept of an Intensive Training and Assessment (ITA) was developed (<www.nhshistopathology.com> 2004).

The ITA programme is a 3-month attachment based at Southampton University Hospital. Trainees spend time in surgical pathology, cytology and autopsy. Towards the end of the 3-month period, they undergo an aptitude assessment similar to that taken by other SHOs. Having successfully completed the assessment, the ITA trainees may apply for SpR posts.

FUTURE STRUCTURE OF HISTOPATHOLOGY TRAINING

The UK Department of Health has recently produced documents under the heading 'Modernising Medical Careers'.[6,7] Far-reaching changes to postgraduate medical education are proposed that will affect all specialties.

All UK graduates from 2005 will undertake a 2-year foundation programme. This will incorporate the current pre-registration year but will provide an additional year of generic clinical training. Proposals have been made for the incorporation of histopathology into the second (F2) year.[8] Various models have been suggested including 4-month full-time attachments, brief one or two week taster courses and clinico-pathological alliances which link histopathology with relevant clinical disciplines.

Initially, it was proposed that foundation programmes would be followed by basic specialty training and higher specialty training. However, it was also suggested that these two components of postgraduate medical education could be amalgamated. This concept has been termed 'run-through training'.[9]

Histopathology is a pilot specialty for run-through training commencing in August 2005. In England, there will be a national recruitment process into the first year of training. Subject to satisfactory progress in the first year, trainees will be allocated to the second and subsequent years of training through a matching scheme. This scheme will take into account personal preferences regarding the location of training.

Trainees will follow a detailed curriculum providing greater guidance than ever before regarding competencies and milestones that must be achieved during the training programme. Progress will be assessed in a variety of ways and will include examinations and work-based assessments.

Subject to approval by the Specialist Training Authority or the Postgraduate Medical Education and Training Board, the minimum length of histopathology training will be reduced from 5.5 years to 5 years (see Fig. 1).

YEAR 1 ASSESSMENT

As appointment to year 1 of training will represent the only competitive hurdle for histopathology trainees, it is essential that a robust assessment of aptitude and progress takes place towards the end of the first year of training. Thus, there will be an RCPath Year 1 Histopathology Assessment taken after 8 months of training with the possibility of a further attempt at 10 months. Trainees who are unsuccessful at the second attempt will receive counselling and it is likely that most will leave the specialty. If there are extenuating circumstances, a trainee may be permitted to repeat year one of training and have a further attempt at the year 1 assessment.

YEARS 2/3

Trainees will undergo at least two years of general histopathology training. The Part 1 MRCPath will be taken during the second or third year and progress to year 4 of training will not be permitted until the Part 1 examination has been passed. The RITA system will be used to extend training for trainees who have not achieved this milestone.

YEARS 3/4

Part 2 MRCPath will be taken during years 3 or 4, depending on experience. Progression to year 5 will not be possible until the Part 2 examination has been passed. Once again, the RITA process will be used to extend training if necessary. This system will allow all trainees at least one year of post-MRCPath training.

YEAR 5

At the end of year 4, assuming that trainees have passed the Part 2 MRCPath, the RITA will take the form of a Penultimate Year Assessment (PYA). This will set goals for year 5 so that trainees can acquire skills that will be relevant to life as a consultant. This may include further training in an area of special interest, management experience and the acquisition of skills in teaching and training. The precise content of the final year of training will depend, to some extent, on the particular career intentions of individual trainees.

INDEPENDENT REPORTING

Prior to the introduction of the SpR grade, senior registrars, and to a lesser extent registrars, in many departments were allowed to issue reports without direct consultant supervision. Following the introduction of the SpR grade, which coincided with a marked decline in the number of trainees in histopathology, this tradition of independent reporting was lost and almost 100% of specimens were directly supervised.

Thus, trainees with 5 years' experience and MRCPath were given virtually no formal responsibility for their work. Many considered this inappropriate in the context of training for consultant practice.

Trainers in Leicester devised a set of graded competencies that would allow trainees to report certain categories of specimens without direct supervision thus re-introducing a more formalised version of the system previously in operation.[10] This fits well with the concept of competency based training that is a major tenet of Modernising Medical Careers. Linkage of the curriculum with independent reporting guidelines will allow trainees to demonstrate the progressive acquisition of relevant competencies.

The issue of graded responsibility has also been considered within American Residency Programmes.[11] In a survey, the authors found that supervising staff and residents in anatomical pathology indicated a willingness to increase the level of independence for residents particularly those of a more senior level. This view has also been supported in the UK.[12]

CONTENT OF HISTOPATHOLOGY TRAINING

Training in histopathology must equip doctors to practice the specialty for 30 years or more. It is, therefore, important to ensure that training is, to some extent, 'future-proofed'. There are several aspects of training that may be subject to change in the short-to-medium term.

THE AUTOPSY

There is at least anecdotal evidence that some doctors are dissuaded from a career in histopathology due to the necessity to train in autopsies. Furthermore, it is likely that the number of autopsies required in future in the UK will diminish.

There has already been a major decline in the hospital autopsy which has been mirrored across the world.[13] In addition, it seems likely that the number of coronial autopsies in England, Wales and Northern Ireland will diminish following recent independent enquires.[14,15] Legislation will be required to introduce the proposed changes that will include an independent review of all deaths. The reviews will be conducted by a medical examiner based in a coroner's office and working outside the National Health Service.[16] Histopathology trainees will need to be aware of these changes in advance of their introduction and to understand the appropriate channels of communication involved.

The RCPath has indicated that it is likely that autopsy-free training will be available within the next few years. However, it will be important to ensure that a cadre of autopsy-trained pathologists remains in order to undertake those autopsies that are required and to perform them to a high standard.

A variety of alternatives to the standard autopsy has been proposed in recent years.[17] These include limited autopsies and needle autopsies, both of which should be familiar to current trainees. These less invasive autopsies may become increasingly common over the next few years, even in coronial cases. Imaging techniques such as angiography and magnetic resonance imaging (MRI) have also been used to undertake post-mortem examinations in adults[18] and neonates.[19] MRI has not only been applied to examination of the intact body but also to perform 'virtual histology' in forensic cases.[20] It remains to be seen who will be responsible for providing reports on such investigations. Will it be radiologists, pathologists, or both? It seems at least possible that histopathology trainees engaged in autopsy practice will require some training in this aspect of post-mortem investigation.

MOLECULAR PATHOLOGY

There have been major developments in the understanding of the molecular basis of disease and the technology available for analysing DNA and RNA. These will undoubtedly lead to a change in pathology practice in the future.

Since histopathologists will be responsible still for the morphological assessment of tissue samples, they should also be encouraged to develop relevant skills in the interpretation of molecular pathology. Thus, it will be important for histopathology training programmes to include education in molecular pathology including an understanding of genetics and the appropriate nucleic acid technology including polymerase chain reaction and gene arrays.[21] In the US, there are now several routes by which nationally recognised certification in molecular pathology can be achieved.[22]

INFORMATICS

The pathologist increasingly needs to be familiar with the concepts of medical informatics. This includes the use of laboratory data systems, including appropriate security measures, the use of statistical packages and internet applications.[23] Many trainees will have perceived computing skills when they enter training. However, self-perception may not always match measured competence. A survey of residents in a pathology training programme in Pittsburgh before and after an informatics course showed that knowledge of informatics improved after the course but that neither pre-test nor post-test scores bore any relation to residents' perceived computer skills.[24]

In the histopathology laboratory of the future, it may be necessary to process complex bio-informatic data as more complex genomic information becomes available. This will require suitable laboratory information systems and appropriately trained pathologists.[25]

DIGITAL MICROSCOPY

High resolution digital imaging is now readily available and has been used as a basis for telepathology and quality assurance schemes. Its use in diagnostic histopathology has been limited but may increase.[28,29]

It is important to prepare trainees for such developments which may impact on their working lives. It is likely, with the availability of rapid high resolution slide scanning, that diagnostic histopathology may be undertaken from digital images on a screen rather than direct microscopy. Even if this technology does not find favour in the diagnostic arena, it is likely to be used more extensively in teaching and training than has been hither to the case.[28,29]

CHANGING WORKFORCE

There have been many changes in the healthcare workforce over recent years. In particular, the role of non-medical staff has been developed and various staff groups have taken on work previously regarded as the province of doctors. There are now nurse practitioners and surgical assistants in clinical practice, in the US and Pathologists' Assistants (PAs) undertake a variety of activities related to surgical pathology and autopsy.[30,31] PAs are highly trained and have been shown to be cost-effective. However, in a survey of pathology residents, a substantial minority of respondents made negative comments about PAs. These comments concerned a perceived adverse impact on resident training and a lack of clarity regarding professional boundaries. Most residents, however, believed that PAs were beneficial as they dealt with simple specimens thus allowing the residents to deal with more complex cases.[32]

These findings are relevant in the UK as the role of biomedical scientists develops. It is now widely accepted that biomedical scientists have a role to play in the examination and sampling of histopathology specimens.[33] When this practice initially came to light, there was some vociferous opposition much of which has now subsided. It will be important to clarify the responsibilities of biomedical staff in relation to medical staff in histopathology, particularly the relationship with medical trainees. There may be shared training for medical and biomedical staff which could help foster mutual understanding.

The introduction of Advanced Practitioners in cytology may also generate uncertainties in the minds of some trainees with respect to professional boundaries. Programme directors will have to ensure that interprofessional working is properly considered during training and will need to emphasise the high level of knowledge and skills required to become an Advanced Practitioner.[34]

PERSONAL AND PROFESSIONAL DEVELOPMENT

There is far more to histopathology training than the development of diagnostic and analytical skills. It is essential that trainees are prepared properly for their professional lives. Even at the outset of a medical career, it may be helpful to obtain some indication of the specialities for which a doctor is suited. For this reason, a speciality choice inventory (Sci45) has been developed in order to help doctors in training choose from a range of specialties that match their attributes and aspirations.[35] The inventory comprises 130 four-response choice items and after its completion will indicate two groups of specialties – one for which the trainee is best suited and one for which they are least suited. This tool could prove helpful at an early stage in training in order to inform career choices by doctors.

Leadership and management skills are increasingly important in the professional lives of pathologists. Management training is difficult to impart by formal didactic lectures and can be difficult to implement within training programmes. A mentor-based approach to leadership and management skills spread throughout a training programme with more intensive training during the final year, has been recommended by some authorities in the US.[36] The most frequently covered topics in US residency programmes were budgets, personnel issues, quality assurance, resource utilisation and equipment evaluation.[37] These topics are equally applicable in the UK.

CONCLUSIONS

Medicine is constantly evolving and histopathology is not exempt from this process. We must be prepared to adapt our training in order to ensure that our trainees are prepared not only for the present but also for the future developments outlined above. Change is inevitable and, in many instances, desirable. Histopathology training must equip doctors with the necessary knowledge, skills and attitudes to practise for 30 years or so. It is essential, therefore, to encourage the flexibility and adaptability that will enhance evolution. The alternative might be extinction.

References

1. Department of Health. *Hospital doctors: training for the future: the report of the working party on specialist medical training (the Calman Report)*. London: Department of Health, 1993.
2. Department of Health. *A guide to specialist registrar training*. London: Department of Health, 1998.
3. Department of Health. *The NHS Cancer plan: a plan for investment, a plan for reform*. London: Department of Health, 2000.
4. Department of Health. *A policy framework for commissioning cancer services: a report by the Expert Advisory Group on Cancer to the Chief Medical Officers of England and Wales – Guidance for providers and purchasers of cancer services*. London: Department of Health, 1999.
5. Gallagher PJ, Dixon MF, Heard S, Moore JK, West KP. An initiative to reform senior house officer training in histopathology. *Hosp Med* 2004; **64**: 303–305.
6. Department of Health. *Modernising medical careers: the response of the four UK Health Ministers to the consultation on 'Unfinished business – proposals for reform of the senior house officer grade'*. London: Department of Health, 2003.
7. Department of Health. *Modernising medical careers: the next steps*. London: Department of Health, 2004.
8. The Royal College of Pathologists. *Modernising medical careers: incorporating pathology into the F2 year*. <http://www.rcpath.org>. Accessed 13 December 2004.
9. Zakhour H, Brinklow J. Run-through training in histopathology. *Bull R Coll Pathol* 2004; **127**: 14–15.
10. The Royal College of Pathologists. *A competency based framework for graded responsibility in histopathology and cytopathology*. London: The Royal College of Pathologists, 2003.
11. Nayar R, Hussong JW. The ASCP resident physician section: results of surveys pertaining to 'graduated responsibility for residents in anatomical pathology'. American Society of Cytopathology. *Am J Clin Pathol* 1997; **107**: 630–631.
12. Evans CA. Nothing becomes real until it is experienced. *Bull R Coll Pathol* 2004; **126**: 18–20.
13. The Royal College of Pathologists of Australasia Autopsy Working Party. The decline of the hospital autopsy: a safety and quality issue for healthcare in Australia. *Med J Aust* 2004; **180**: 281–285.
14. HMSO. *Death certification and investigation in England Wales and Northern Ireland: results of a fundamental review*. Cm5831. London: HMSO, 2003.
15. HMSO. *The Shipman inquiry third report: death certification and the investigation of deaths by coroners*. Cm5854. London: HMSO, 2003.
16. Hasleton P. Reforming the coroner and death certification service. *Curr Diagn Pathol* 2004; **10**: 453–462.
17. Benbow EW, Roberts IS. The autopsy: complete or not? *Histopathology* 2003; **42**: 417–423.
18. Bisset RAL, Thomas B, Turnbull W, Lee S. Post-mortem examinations using magnetic resonance imaging: four year review of a working service. *BMJ* 2002; **324**: 1423–1424.
19. Huisman TA. Magnetic resonance imaging: an alternative to autopsy in neonatal death? *Semin Neonatol* 2004; **9**: 347–353.
20. Thali MJ, Dimhofer R, Becker R, Oliver W, Potter K. Is 'virtual histology' the next step in the 'virtual autopsy'? Magnetic resonance microscopy in forensic medicine. *Magn Reson Imaging* 2004; **8**: 1131–1138.
21. The Association for Molecular Pathology Training and Education Committee. Goals and objectives for molecular training in residency programs. *J Mol Diagn* 1999; **1**: 5–15.
22. Killeen AA, Wai-Choi L, Payne D *et al*. Certification in molecular pathology in the

United States (Training and Education Committee, the Association for Molecular Pathology). *J Mol Diagn* 2002; **4**: 181–184.

23. Henricks WH, Boyer PJ, Harrison JH *et al*. Informatics training in pathology residency programs: proposed learning objectives and skill sets for the new millenium. *Arch Pathol Lab Med* 2003; **127**: 1009–1018.

24. Harrison JH, Stewart J. Training in pathology informatics: implementation at the University of Pittsburgh. *Arch Pathol Lab Med* 2003; **127**: 1019–1025.

25. Becich MJ. The role of the pathologist as tissue refiner and data miner: the impact of functional genomics on the modern pathology laboratory and the critical roles of pathology informatics and bioinformatics. *Mol Diagn* 2000; **5**: 287–299.

26. O'Brien MJ, Sotnikov AV. Digital imaging in anatomic pathology. *Am J Clin Pathol* 1996; **106 (4 Suppl)**: S25–S32.

27. Felten CL, Strauss JS, Okada DH, Marchevsky AM. Virtual microscopy: high resolution digital photomicrography, a tool for light microscopy simulation. *Hum Pathol* 1999; **30**: 477–483.

28. Kumar R, Velan GM, Korell SO *et al*. Virtual microscopy for learning and assessment. *J Pathol* 2004; **204**: 613–618.

29. Lundin M, Lundin J, Helin H, Isola J. A digital atlas of breast histopathology: an application of web based virtual microscopy. *J Clin Pathol* 2004; **57**: 1288–1291.

30. Grzybicki DM, Reilly TL, Hart AR *et al*. National practice characteristics and utilisation of pathologists' assistants. *Arch Pathol Lab Med* 2001; **125**: 905–912.

31. Grzybicki DM, Vrbin CM, Reilly TL *et al*. Use of physician extenders in surgical pathology practice. *Arch Pathol Lab Med* 2003; **128**:165–172.

32. Grzybicki DM, Vrbin CM. Pathology residents' attitudes and opinions about pathologists' assistants. *Arch Pathol Lab Med* 2003; **127**: 666–672.

33. Duthie FR, Nairn ER, Milne AW *et al*. The impact of involvement of biomedical scientists in specimen dissection and selection of blocks for histopathology: a study of time benefits and specimen handling quality in Ayrshire and Arran area laboratory. *J Clin Pathol* 2004; **57**: 27–32.

34. Smith PA, Hewer EM. Examination for the certificate in advanced practice in cervical cytology – the first year's experience. *Cytopathology* 2003; **14**: 101–104.

35. Gale R, Grant J. Sci45: the development of a specialty choice inventory. *Med Educ* 2002; 36: 659–666.

36. Sims KL, Darcy TP. A leadership-management training curriculum for pathology residents. *Am J Clin Pathol* 1997; **108**: 90–95.

37. Goldberg-Kahn B, Sims KL, Darcy TP. Survey of management training in United States and Canadian pathology residency programs. *Am J Clin Pathol* 1997; **108**: 96–100.

Jeffrey S. Ross

3

Predictive and prognostic molecular markers in breast cancer

Substantial progress has been made over the past three decades in our understanding of the epidemiology, clinical course and basic biology of breast cancer.[1] Tangible changes have occurred in areas of early detection, risk assessment and combined modality treatment that have transformed our ability to manage and, in many cases, cure breast cancer. Morphology has been the cornerstone for the characterisation of breast cancer prognosis.[2] Tumour type, grade, size, lymph node status, and overall pathological stage comprise critical factors used to assess the risk of breast cancer progression after diagnosis. Additional morphology-based assessments used to assess prognosis include: extent of *in-situ* carcinoma component, resection margin status, lymphovascular invasion, microvessel density, tumour infiltrating lymphocytes, skin involvement and the presence of Paget's disease.[3] This chapter considers the existing ancillary tests and emerging molecular markers in breast cancer prognosis assessment and the prediction of response of breast cancer to treatment of the disease.

CURRENT PRACTICE

Ancillary prognostic and predictive factors in current practice are illustrated in Figure 1.

HORMONE RECEPTOR STATUS

The role of oestrogen (ER) and progesterone (PR) receptor testing as markers of prognosis and predictors of response to anti-oestrogen therapy is

Jeffrey S. Ross MD
Cyrus Strong Merrill Professor and Chair, Department of Pathology and Laboratory Medicine,
Albany Medical College MC-80, 47 New Scotland Avenue, Albany, NY 12208, USA
(E-mail: rossj@mail.amc.edu)
Division of Oncology Molecular Medicine, Millennium Pharmaceuticals, Inc., Cambridge,
Massachusetts, USA

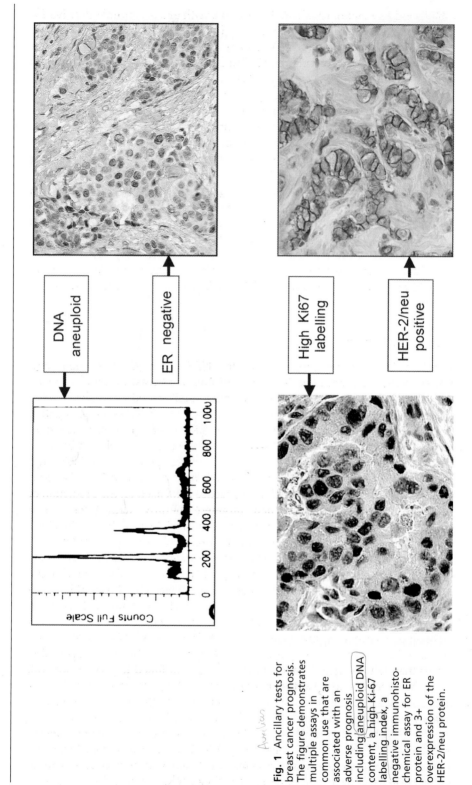

Fig. 1 Ancillary tests for breast cancer prognosis. The figure demonstrates multiple assays in common use that are associated with an adverse prognosis including aneuploid DNA content, a high Ki-67 labelling index, a negative immunohistochemical assay for ER protein and 3+ overexpression of the HER-2/neu protein.

established as a standard of care for patients with breast cancer.[4,5] Positive ER and PR assays are associated with well-differentiated histology, negative lymph node status, diploid DNA content, low cell proliferation rate and the tendency for a relatively indolent clinical course.[4-6] ER/PR-negative tumours are often associated with aggressive disease including amplification of the HER-2/*neu*, C-*myc* and *int-2* oncogenes, mutation of the *p-53* gene, and up-regulation of invasion- and metastasis-associated growth factors, growth factor receptors and proteases.[4,5] The determination of ER/PR status in newly diagnosed breast cancer is required for selection of patients to receive hormonal therapy and the ER/PR has also been widely used to predict risk for progressive disease.[6] Originally determined on fresh tumour protein extracts and cytosols using a quantitative biochemical competitive binding assay with dextran-coated charcoal, the small size of newly diagnosed primary tumours has required a shift to on-slide immunohistochemical methods.[7] Despite its limitations including the lack of standardisation, immunohistochemistry is currently the standard method to determine ER and PR status in breast cancer; in addition, it remains a cornerstone of planning of therapy for the disease and appears to be likely to be utilised clinically in this fashion for the foreseeable future.

HER-2/*neu* STATUS

Amplification and overexpression of the HER-2/*neu* (C-*erb*B-2) gene and protein have been identified in 10–34% of invasive breast cancers.[8] The vast majority of these studies have linked either gene amplification or protein overexpression of HER-2/*neu* with adverse prognosis in either node-negative or node-positive disease.[8] In general, when specimens have been carefully fixed, processed and embedded, there has been excellent correlation between gene copy status determined by fluorescence *in-situ* hybridisation (FISH) and protein expression levels determined by immunohistochemically.[8] The main use of either method in current clinical practice is focused on the prediction of response to the anti-HER-2/neu targeted therapy with trastuzumab (Herceptin™).[8] For this reason, the American Society of Clinical Oncology (ASCO) and the College of American Pathologists (CAP) both consider HER-2/neu testing to be part of the standard work-up for a newly diagnosed breast cancer specimen.[9,10] Recently, the chromogenic *in-situ* hybridisation technique has been applied to breast cancer specimens to determine their HER-2/neu status with promising results (Fig. 2).[11] Molecular techniques have been assessed for their ability to out-perform slide-based assays. The RT-PCR technique,[12,13] predominantly used to detect HER-2/*neu* mRNA in peripheral blood and bone marrow samples, has correlated more with gene amplification status than with immunohistochemical levels,[14] but failed to predict survival. With the advent of laser-capture microscopy and the acceptance of RT-PCR as a routine and reproducible laboratory technique, its role in HER-2/*neu* status assessment may increase in the future. The cDNA microarray-based method of detecting HER-2/*neu* mRNA expression levels has recently achieved interest as an alternative method for measuring HER-2/*neu* status in breast cancer.[15] This method has the advantage of being able to assess downstream signalling of the HER-2 and other pathways such as ER at the same time that the level of

HER-2 mRNA is measured. In a recent study, the HER-2/*neu* gene amplification status detected by FISH on 20 paraffin-embedded breast cancer core biopsy samples was correctly predicted in all cases by the quantification of the HER-2 mRNA levels obtained by expression profiling of mRNA extracted from paired fine needle aspiration biopsies from the same patients.[15] A summary of HER-2/neu testing methods ion breast cancer is shown in Table 1.

DNA PLOIDY AND S PHASE

Studies on the prognostic significance of DNA content analysis (DNA ploidy) and S-phase status have varied greatly with some investigators finding significant prediction of disease-free and overall survival on both univariate and multivariate analysis and others finding no impact on disease outcome.[16] The S phase calculation by flow cytometry has generally out-performed ploidy status as a prognostic factor in breast cancer and is advocated by some investigators as a useful clinical parameter. Despite their continuing clinical use in many institutions, neither ASCO[9] nor CAP[10] include ploidy and S-phase measurements in their lists of recommended prognostic factors. The lack of a standardised approach to performing this test and interpreting its result is the major reason S phase fraction is not accepted as a standard prognostic marker.

Ki-67 LABELLING

Cell proliferation labelling measured by Ki-67 immunostaining correlates with the S-phase levels calculated by flow cytometry, but is generally higher

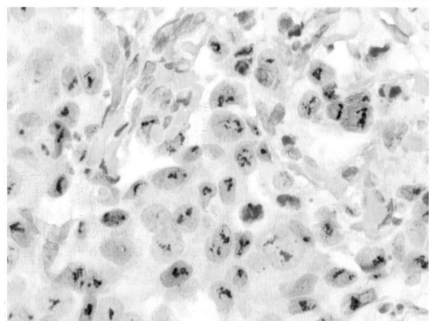

Fig. 2 HER-2/*neu* gene amplification in infiltrating breast cancer detected by chromogenic *in-situ* hybridisation (CISH) using anti-HER-2/*neu* probe and immunohistochemistry with diaminobenzidine chromagen (SpotLight™ HER-2/*neu* probe, Zymed Corp., South San Francisco, CA, USA).

Table 1 Summary of HER-2/neu testing methods

TEST	IHC	FISH	CISH	Tumour ELISA	RT-PCR	Expression profiling
Substance tested	Protein	DNA	DNA	Protein	mRNA	mRNA
Typical sample type	FFPE	FFPE	FFPE	Fresh cytosol Protein extract	Fresh Frozen	Fresh Frozen
Suitable for FNA	No	Yes	Yes	No	Yes	Yes
Degree of quantitation	Semi-quantitative Image analysis of slides is more quantitative	Quantitative	Semi-quantitative Difficult to count gene copies in 3–6 copies/cell range or when count is greater than 8 copies/cell	Quantitative Uses standard curve and reports in absolute units of HER-2/neu protein	Semi-quantitative Relative gene expression score compared to standard house-keeping genes	Semi-quantitative Relative gene expression score compared to standard house-keeping genes
FDA status	Approved for predicting trastuzumab response	Approved for predicting trastuzumab response	Not approved	Not approved (serum ELISA is approved)	Not approved	Not approved
Estimated cost/test (technical reagents only in US$)	Non-FDA approved: $7–11. FDA-approved: $25–40	Non-FDA approved: $25–35. FDA-approved: $40–80	Non-FDA approved: $20–35	Non-FDA approved: $30–45	Non-FDA approved: $40–55	Non-FDA approved: $200–500
Comment	Most prevalent technique in clinical practice. Slide scoring difficulties are reduced by the use of image analysis	May out-perform IHC for predicting trastuzumab response	Combines advantages of IHC and FISH while avoiding cost of fluorescence microscope	Excellent performance, but requires fresh protein cytosol/extract which limits test to larger resected primary tumours only	mRNA expression correlates with DNA copy number and protein expression	Currently an expensive approach, but offers both multiplex data on other prognostic and pharmacogenomic markers and downstream pathway activation information

FFPE, formalin-fixed paraffin-embedded tissue sections; IHC, immunohistochemistry; FISH, fluorescence *in-situ* hybridisation; CISH, chromogenic *in-situ* hybridisation; ELISA, enzyme linked immunosorbent assay; RT-PCR, real time polymerase chain reaction; FDA, US Food and Drug Administration reflecting the fact that the Ki-67 antigen is also expressed in late G_1 as well early G_2/M phases of the cell cycle.[17] Ki-67 staining has achieved a more consistent significant correlation with breast cancer outcome both on univariate and multivariate analysis than DNA ploidy alone. However, this test despite being easily performed on formalin-fixed, paraffin-embedded tissue sections, suffers from the lack of standardisation including the general lack of use of cell line controls of known proliferative index.

RESEARCH-ORIENTED TESTS OCCASIONALLY USED IN CLINICAL PRACTICE

CELL CYCLE MARKERS

Amplification or overexpression of cyclin D1 (*PRAD1*; bcl-1), localised to chromosome 11q13 has also been identified in 20% of clinical breast cancers[18] and has been linked to the expression of the oestrogen receptor[19] and the transition from *in-situ* to invasive ductal breast cancer.[20] In a recent study, high levels of the low-molecular-weight isoforms of cyclin E, measured by Western blotting, correlated strongly with decreased disease-specific survival;[21] moreover, levels of total cyclin E also were highly correlative with poor outcome consistent with prior studies performed by immunohistochemistry.[22] The p21 protein (p21/WAF1/Cip1) is an inhibitor of cyclin-dependent kinases and serves as a critical downstream effector in the p53-specific pathway of cell growth control.[23] Some studies have linked altered expression of p21 with adverse outcome in breast cancer,[24,25] whereas others have not.[26] p27 (kip1) is a cell-cycle regulator that acts by binding and inactivating cyclin-dependent kinases.[26] Low p27 expression has been correlated with poor prognosis in many (but not all) studies of patients especially with small primary tumours.[27–30]

ONCOGENES

The measurement of oncogene activity has not played a major role in the clinical assessment of breast cancer specimens to date. The C-*myc* gene is amplified in about 16% of breast cancer cases and, in the majority of outcome-based studies, is associated with decreased disease-free patient survival.[31] In addition, overexpression of the N-*myc* oncogene has also been associated with tumour grade, stage and adverse prognosis.[32] The H-*ras* gene has been consistently associated with breast cancer progression.[33,34] Measurements of the c-*fos* (chromosome14q21) and c-*jun* (chromosome 22q13) regulators of the activating protein-1(AP-1) complex and c-*myb* (chromosome 6q21) have successfully predicted breast cancer recurrence, response to hormonal therapy and survival.[35]

*p*53 AND TUMOUR SUPPRESSOR GENES

The prognostic significance of p53 status in breast cancer has been impacted by the accuracy of immunohistochemical versus molecular methods (SSCP, direct sequencing and the yeast colony functional assay).[36,37] The *p53* mutation rate is lower in breast cancer than in other carcinomas and has been associated with progressive disease and reduced overall survival.[38–40] In general, breast carcinomas with *p53* mutations are associated with high histological grade, high mitotic index, high cell proliferation rate, aneuploid DNA content, negative assays for oestrogen and progesterone receptor[41] and variable association with amplification of oncogenes such as HER-2/*neu*, C-*myc*, *ras*, and *int-2*.[42] Some, but not all, studies have implicated *p53* mutation with resistance to hormonal, adjuvant and neo-adjuvant chemotherapy and combination chemotherapy for metastatic disease encompassing a variety of agents, including anthracyclines and taxanes.[43–51] Currently, determination of p53 status is not included as a part of the standard of practice for the management of breast cancer. Other tumour suppressor genes such as *Rb* have not been widely applied to breast cancer although a recent study of the E2F1 transcription factor which is activated when *Rb* is suppressed showed significant prognostic impact for this marker in patients treated with multi-agent cytotoxic drugs.[52]

CELL ADHESION MOLECULES

Cell adhesion molecule expression has been extensively studied in breast cancer as a biomarker of tumour development, differentiation, progression and metastasis.[53,54] The E-cadherin–catenin complex has been related to disease outcome in a variety of malignant diseases including breast cancer.[55] The majority of published studies have linked loss of expression of E-cadherin with adverse outcome in breast cancer,[56–58] although there have been reports of retained expression indicating disease progression.[59] The most consistent observation concerning the loss of E-cadherin expression in breast cancer has been the association with the infiltrating lobular pattern versus infiltrating ductal pattern of invasive carcinoma.[60–62] E-cadherin status has not been widely used to predict the response of breast cancer to therapy. CD44 expression has been associated with the development and progression of breast cancer.[63] Abnormal expression of the standard form of CD44 has been linked to prognosis.[64] Overexpression of the CD44 splice variant v6 has been linked to adverse outcome in several studies,[65–67] but not in others.[68] The integrin group and laminin receptor group have been widely studied in breast cancer.[69] Laminin receptor expression has been independently associated with disease outcome in some studies,[70,71] but not in others.[72] Altered expression of integrins αv[73] and $\alpha 6$[74,75] have been linked to breast cancer prognosis.

bcl-2 AND APOPTOSIS

In breast cancer, the majority of studies have linked an increased rate of cellular apoptosis with an adverse outcome for the disease.[76–79] Expression of the anti-apoptosis-associated gene *Bcl-2* correlates with ER/PR-positive status and has been associated with improved patient survival.[80–82] In one study, bcl-2 expression has been linked to prognosis in tamoxifen-treated breast cancer, but not in patients treated with surgery alone.[83] However, primary tumour bcl-2 expression levels have not been predictive for response to systemic chemotherapy given after relapse.[84] Expression of the pro-apoptosis gene *Bax* has not been clearly linked to outcome.[85] In addition, activated caspases can act as both initiators and effectors of the apoptotic pathway and there is evidence that caspases 3, 6, and 8 are associated with higher levels of apoptosis, histological grade and tumour aggressiveness in breast cancer.[86] Caspase expression in breast cancer has been linked to overall survival[87] and chemoresistance.[88]

INVASION-ASSOCIATED PROTEASES

Numerous studies in the early 1990s using an immunoassay approach on fresh breast tumour cytosolic preparations have shown that elevated cathepsin D levels are an independent predictor of survival in breast cancer.[89–91] Attempts to convert the assay to an immunohistochemical-based format have not been successful.[92,93] The serine proteases studied in breast cancer invasion have focused on urokinase plasminogen activator, receptor and plasminogen activator inhibitor-1 (uPA, uPAR and PAI-1). When evaluated on fresh tissue extracts and tumour cytosols, high uPA and PAI-1 levels have been consistently associated with disease recurrence and overall patient survival in breast cancer.[94–97] Translation of the uPA/PAI-1 immunoassay to an on-slide immunohistochemical format has not, to date, been successful; this has limited wide-spread use. The matrix metalloproteases (MMPs) are a group of at least 19 zinc metallo-enzymes secreted as pro-enzymes with substantial sequence similarities that are inhibited by metallochelators and specific tissue inhibitors known as TIMPs.[98] The MMPs include the interstitial collagenases, gelatinases, stromelysins and membrane-type MMPs and are involved in breast cancer initiation, invasion and metastasis.[98] High levels of at least three MMPs (MMP-2, MMP-9 and MMP-11) have been found to correlate with poor disease outcome in breast cancer.[99–101]

VEGF AND ANGIOGENESIS MARKERS

In breast cancer, most of the studies addressing the clinical relevance of angiogenic factors to predict the course of the disease have centred on VEGF and associated factors.[102] A significant number of studies have implicated high levels of VEGF in patient serum, in tumour protein extracts and in tumour tissues using immunohistochemistry as an adverse prognostic factor for both node-negative and node-positive disease.[103–105] These studies have also been linked to the presence of increased microvessel density in breast tumours conveying an adverse prognosis.

EMERGING PROGNOSTIC AND PREDICTIVE FACTORS

ONCOTYPE DX

The Oncotype Dx is an RT-PCR multiplex assay using a 21-gene probe set and mRNA extracted from paraffin blocks of stored breast cancer tissues.[106] Using a cohort of 688 lymph node negative; ER+ tumours obtained from patients enrolled in two NSABP clinical trials treated with tamoxifen alone, the 21-gene assay predicted disease recurrence to a high level of significance ($P < 0.00001$).[106] This assay has recently become available for new patients.

Whole genome transcriptional profiling has been used as a technique for the classification[107] of breast cancer and for determining its prognosis.[108–110] Gene expression profiles can define cellular functions, biochemical pathways, cell proliferation activity and regulatory mechanisms. In a DNA microarray analysis on primary breast tumours of 117 node-negative young patients using a supervised classification to identify a poor prognosis gene expression signature, aberrant expression of genes regulating cell cycle, invasion, metastasis and angiogenesis strongly predicted a short interval to distant metastases.[109] In a follow-up study, the poor prognosis gene expression profile outperformed all currently used clinical parameters in predicting disease outcome including lymph node status with an estimated hazard ratio for distant metastases of 5.1 (95% confidence interval, 2.9–9.0; $P < 0.001$).[110] DNA microarrays addressing cancer outcomes show variable prognostic performance. Larger studies with appropriate clinical design, adjustment for known predictors, and proper validation are essential for this highly promising technology.[111]

The hierarchical clustering technique of data analysis from transcriptional profiling of clinical samples known to have responded or been resistant to a single agent or combination of anti-cancer drugs (Fig. 3) has recently been employed as a guide to anticancer drug therapy in cancers of the breast and other organs.[112] Using transcriptional profiling, the microarray technique has been able to generate an 81% accuracy for predicting the presence or absence of pathological complete response after pre-operative chemotherapy with sequential weekly paclitaxel and 5-fluorouracil, doxorubicin and cyclophosphamide (FAC) in breast cancer.[112] More importantly, 75% of the patients who were predicted to have complete pathological response based on their gene expression profile indeed experienced complete response. This compares very favourably with the 25–30% chance of complete response that unselected patients may expect with this treatment regimen. Using commercial oligonucleotide microarrays with the mRNA extracted from core needle biopsies, a recent report found that different patterns of gene expression significantly correlated with docetaxel response in breast cancer.[113]

The potential of pharmacogenomics as a novel tool for identifying clinically important subgroups of patients is enormous. However, the challenges that need to be solved before routine clinical application are also significant. A very important challenge is standardisation. Currently, multiple microarray platforms exist that use distinct sets of genes and employ different hybridisation and signal detection methods. Some arrays contain cDNAs of variable length while others contain small oligonucleotide sequences. In different oligonucleotide arrays, the same gene may be represented by different sequences. Furthermore, investigators that utilise competitive hybridisation between fluorescein-labelled biological samples and a standard control sample invariably use different controls from laboratory to laboratory. Not surprisingly, marker sets generated by one laboratory differ significantly from marker sets generated by others for the same purpose. Furthermore, the type of tissue sampling clearly has a major impact on profiling results since the transcriptional profiles are a composite of mRNA contributed by all tissue

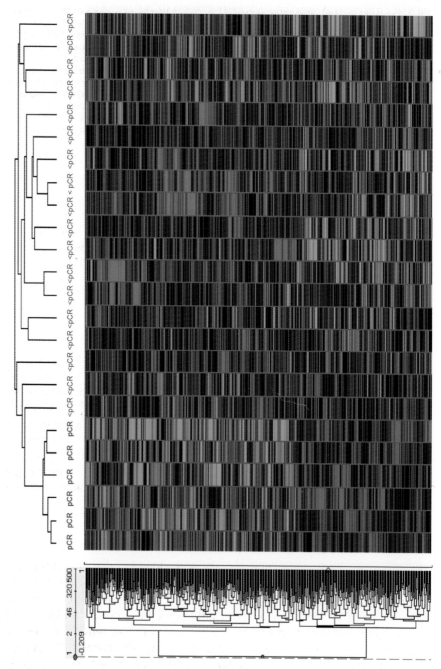

Fig. 3 (See caption at top of next page)

components of the biological sample. Microdissected tissue, fine needle aspiration or core needle biopsy will all give a significantly different transcriptional profile from the same cancer. In brief, results generated by one group of investigators may only be valid to the DNA microarray platform and tissue sampling technique that is used in that particular laboratory. Interpretation of microarray results is also very different from interpretation of

Fig. 3 (*See opposite page*) Gene expression profiling of fine needle aspirations of breast cancer identifies genes associated with complete pathological response to neoadjuvant taxol/FAC chemotherapy. Supervised clustering of the top 500 SNR markers associated with pathological response from the 24 training samples. All the pathological complete responders (pCR) cluster together and are separated from the samples that had incomplete pathological response (<pCR). In this study, an 81% accuracy of predicting the presence or absence of pathological complete response after pre-operative chemotherapy with sequential weekly paclitaxel and 5-fluorouracil, doxorubicin and cyclophosphamide (FAC) in breast cancer was achieved. More importantly, 75% of the patients who were predicted to have complete pathological response based on their gene expression profile indeed experienced complete response. This compares very favourably with the 25–30% chance of complete response that unselected patients typically expect with this treatment

conventional prognostic markers. Immunohistochemistry for ER can be performed by any number of antibodies that recognise the ER protein and the staining can be interpreted similarly by any well-trained pathologist. In contrast, microarray profiles only make sense in the context of other profiles. The profiling result must be compared with a pre-existing database of profiles to make a prediction. Furthermore, the predictive precision will increase as the database increases, which also implies that the marker set will undergo revisions periodically to fit observed clinical outcomes better.

PROTEOMICS

MALDI and SELDI mass spectrometry and other proteomics' strategies have shown preliminary success for the early detection of ovarian cancer[114] and have recently been applied to breast cancer for the discovery of new and better biomarkers both in serum and nipple aspirate specimens.[115,116] Although further testing of this approach must be performed on larger groups of patients, the SELDI-TOF technique shows promise as a potential method of developing new disease markers capable of detecting cancers at early stages. However, most studies using mass spectroscopy and two-dimensional gel electrophoresis have utilised breast cancer cell lines in preclinical models and have not, to date, been widely translated to clinical specimens.

CIRCULATING TUMOUR CELLS

The discovery of circulating tumour cells in the blood of patients with breast cancer came at a relatively early phase of the broadening of research in the disease.[117] Peripheral blood cell capture techniques often employ immunomagnetic beads coated with antibodies to epithelial antigens and glycoproteins expressed on the surface of the malignant cells. In a recently published prospective multicentre study involving 177 patients with proven metastatic breast cancer who were starting a new line of treatment, the levels of circulating tumour cells at baseline and at the first follow-up visit were the most significant predictors of progression-free and overall survival.[118]

DNA METHYLATION

The detection of methylated DNA accompanied by the silencing of the effected genes has emerged as a novel approach for the detection of cancer in blood and

Table 2 Ancillary/molecular prognostic factors in breast cancer

Biomarker	Assay	Target of therapy	Therapeutic	Current status	Future prospects
ER/PR	IHC binding assay	Yes	Tamoxifen, SERMs, aromatase inhibitors	Standard of care	Improved IHC with antibodies that are negative when ERα is truncated to reduce false positives
HER-2/neu	IHC, FISH	Yes	Herceptin, other anti-bodies, gene therapy	Standard of care	CISH assay may replace both IHC and FISH
DNA ploidy	Cytometry	No	–	Common use	Decreased use
S phase	Cytometry	No	–	Common use	Maintained use
Thymidine labelling index	Radioactive [³H]-thymidine incorporation during DNA synthesis	No	–	Rarely used	Decreased use due to methodological barrier. Has yielded to the Ki-67 labelling index (below)
Ki-67 labelling index	IHC	No	–	Widely used	Continued expansion as replacement of the S phase measurement by flow cytometry
Cyclin D	IHC	Possible	Flavopyridol, translocation targets	Clinical trials	May select new drug use such as proteasome inhibitors
Cyclin E	IHC, Western	No	–	RUO	Prognostic significance must be validated
EGFR	IHC, FISH	Yes	Iressa, tarceva, erbitux	Increasing use, clinical trials	Targeting the anti-EGFR drugs likely combined with pharmacogenomics
VEGF	IHC	Yes	Avastin, small molecules	Increasing use, clinical trials	Increasing use for prognosis. Initial targeted therapy disappointing
p53	IHC, SSCP sequencing	Yes	Gene therapy	Increasing use, clinical trials	Targeted therapies disappointing to date
E-cadherin	IHC, methylation-PCR	Yes	5-azacytidine demethylation	Increasing use, clinical trials	Diagnosis of pleomorphic lobular carcinoma

Table 2 (continued) Ancillary/molecular prognostic factors in breast cancer

Biomarker	Assay	Target of therapy	Therapeutic	Current status	Future prospects
CD-44 v6	IHC	No	–	RUO	Predictive significance of v6 splice variant requires validation
Cathepsin D	Immunoassay	No	–	Common use in Europe	IHC studies disappointing; will continue to fade from view
uPA/PAI-1	Immunoassay	Yes	Small molecules (e.g. WX-UK1)	Common use in Europe	Targeted therapies in early stages. IHC assays not validated to date restricting use in the US
MMPs 2, 9, 11	IHC	Yes	Marmistat	Clinical trials, RUO	Early results of targeted therapy disappointing
MDR	IHC	Yes	Small molecules	Clinical trials, RUO	Continued use
Bcl-2	IHC	Yes	Genasense, proteasome inhibitors	Increasing use, clinical trials	Initial results of targeted therapies disappointing
Telomerase	TRAP, IHC, ISH	Yes	Small molecules	RUO	Increased use if slide-based assays are successful prognostic factors
NF-κB	IHC, Western	Yes	Proteasome inhibitors	RUO	Will be used if targeted therapies are successful alone or in combination with cytotoxic drugs
Oncotype DX	RT-PCR (paraffin)	No	–	RUO	Recent study of 668 node negative, ER+ cases treated with tamoxifen only showed 21 gene RT-PCR expression assay could predict risk of disease recurrence at $P < 0.00001$
Transcriptional profiling	cDNA array, oligonucleotide array	No	–	RUO	Continued major expansion of use. Predictive marker sets will require multiple cross-validation. Could become standard if initial results are confirmed

SSCP, single strand conformation polymorphism; RUO, research use only; WK-UK1, Wilex, Inc., Munich, Germany.

body fluids.[119] DNA methylation assays have been applied to nipple duct aspirates in an attempt to detect breast cancer at an early stage.[119] The assessment of DNA methylation as a prognostic factor for breast cancer has only recently been carried out. In a study of 86 patients using a broad-spectrum, serum-based DNA methylation assay, multivariate analysis showed that methylation of two genes, *RASSF1A* and/or *APC* were independently associated with poor clinical outcome of the disease.[120] Further studies of DNA methylation and other epigenetic phenomena in circulation are currently being tested for their potential to guide therapy for breast cancer.

Points for best practice

- The search for more accurate prognostic tests and tests designed to predict response to therapy for breast cancer will continue to challenge scientists and clinicians.

- A variety of emerging molecular diagnostic tests are continually being introduced for breast cancer management (Table 2).

- The most useful prognostic/predictive factors are hormone receptor status and HER-2/*neu* status and are likely to remain the principal ancillary tests of invasive breast cancer specimens for the foreseeable future.

- Gene expression profiling performed by either RT-PCR or DNA microarray methods are likely to compete with proteomic strategies in the development of both prognostic and predictive tests designed to individualise treatment and further fulfil the promise of a truly personalised treatment for breast cancer patients.

References

1. Jemal A, Murray T, Samuels A *et al*. Cancer statistics. *Cancer J Clin* 2003; **53**: 5–26.
2. Fitzgibbons PL, Page DL, Weaver D *et al* Prognostic factors in breast cancer. College of American Pathologists Consensus Statement 1999. *Arch Pathol Lab Med* 2000; **124**: 966–978.
3. Ross JS, Linette GP, Stec J *et al*. Breast cancer biomarkers and molecular medicine. *Expert Rev Mol Diagn* 2003; **3**: 573–585.
4. Osborne CK. Steroid hormone receptors in breast cancer management. *Breast Cancer Res Treat* 1998; **51**: 227–238.
5. Locker GY. Hormonal therapy of breast cancer. *Cancer Treat Rev* 1998; **24**: 221–240.
6. Bertucci F, Houlgatte R, Benziane A *et al*. Gene expression profiling of primary breast carcinomas using arrays of candidate genes. *Hum Mol Genet* 2000; **9**: 2981–2991.
7. Masood S. Prediction of recurrence for advanced breast cancer. Traditional and contemporary pathologic and molecular markers. *Surg Oncol Clin North Am* 1995; **4**: 601–632.
8. Ross JS, Fletcher JA, Linette GP *et al*. The Her-2/*neu* gene and protein in breast cancer 2003: biomarker and target of therapy. *Oncologist* 2003; **8**: 307–325.
9. Bast Jr RC, Ravdin P, Hayes DF *et al*. 2000 update of recommendations for the use of tumor markers in breast and colorectal cancer: clinical practice guidelines of the American Society of Clinical Oncology. *J Clin Oncol* 2001; **19**: 1865–1878.
10. Hammond ME, Fitzgibbons PL, Compton CC *et al*. College of American Pathologists Conference XXXV: solid tumor prognostic factors-which, how and so what? Summary

document and recommendations for implementation. Cancer Committee and Conference Participants. *Arch Pathol Lab Med* 2000; **124**: 958–965.

11. Dandachi N, Dietze O, Hauser-Kronberger C. Evaluation of the clinical significance of HER2 amplification by chromogenic in situ hybridisation in patients with primary breast cancer. *Anticancer Res* 2004; **24**: 2401–2406.

12. Pawlowski V, Revillion F, Hornez L *et al*. A real-time one-step reverse transcriptase-polymerase chain reaction method to quantify c-erbB-2 expression in human breast cancer. *Cancer Detect Prev* 2000; **24**: 212–223.

13. Bieche I, Onody P, Laurendeau I *et al*. Real-time reverse transcription-PCR assay for future management of ERBB2-based clinical applications. *Clin Chem* 1999; **45**: 1148–1156.

14. Tubbs RR, Pettay JD, Roche PC *et al*. Discrepancies in clinical laboratory testing of eligibility for trastuzumab therapy: apparent immunohistochemical false-positives do not get the message. *J Clin Oncol* 2001; **19**: 2714–2721.

15. Pusztai L, Ayers M, Stec J *et al*. Gene expression profiles obtained from fine-needle aspirations of breast cancer reliably identify routine prognostic markers and reveal large-scale molecular differences between estrogen-negative and estrogen-positive tumors. *Clin Cancer Res* 2003; **9**: 2406–2415.

16. Ross, JS. *DNA ploidy and Cell Cycle Analysis in Pathology*. New York: Igaku-Shoin, 1996; 54–55.

17. MacGrogan G, Jollet I, Huet S *et al*. Comparison of quantitative and semiquantitative methods of assessing MIB-1 with the S-phase fraction in breast carcinoma. *Modern Pathol* 1997; **10**: 769–776.

18. Wolman SR, Pauley RJ, Mohamed AN *et al*. Genetic markers as prognostic indicators in breast cancer. *Cancer* 1992; **70**: 1765–1774.

19. Steeg PS, Zhou Q. Cyclins and breast cancer. *Breast Cancer Res Treat* 1998; **52**: 17–28.

20. Weinstat-Saslow D, Merino MJ, Manrow RE *et al*. Overexpression of cyclin D mRNA distinguishes invasive and in situ breast carcinomas from non-malignant lesions. *Nat Med* 1995; **1**: 1257–1260.

21. Keyomarsi K, Tucker SL, Buchholz TA *et al*. Cyclin E and survival in patients with breast cancer. *N Engl J Med* 2002; **347**: 1566–1575.

22. Keyomarsi K, O'Leary N, Molnar G *et al*. Cyclin E, a potential prognostic marker for breast cancer. *Cancer Res* 1994; **54**: 380–385.

23. Caffo O, Doglioni C, Veronese S *et al*. Prognostic value of p21(WAF1) and p53 expression in breast carcinoma: an immunohistochemical study in 261 patients with long-term follow-up. *Clin Cancer Res* 1996; **2**: 1591–1599.

24. Oh YL, Choi JS, Song SY *et al*. Expression of p21Waf1, p27Kip1 and cyclin D1 proteins in breast ductal carcinoma *in situ*: relation with clinicopathologic characteristics and with p53 expression and estrogen receptor status. *Pathol Int* 2001; **51**: 94–99.

25. Gohring UJ, Bersch A, Becker M *et al*. p21(waf) correlates with DNA replication but not with prognosis in invasive breast cancer. *J Clin Pathol* 2001; 54: 866–870.

26. Lau R, Grimson R, Sansome C *et al*. Low levels of cell cycle inhibitor p27kip1 combined with high levels of Ki-67 predict shortened disease-free survival in T1 and T2 invasive breast carcinomas. *Int J Oncol* 2001; **18**: 17–23.

27. Barbareschi M. p27 expression, a cyclin dependent kinase inhibitor in breast carcinoma. *Adv Clin Pathol* 1999; **20**: 119–127.

28. Barbareschi M, van Tinteren H, Mauri FA *et al*. p27(kip1) expression in breast carcinomas: an immunohistochemical study on 512 patients with long-term follow-up. *Int J Cancer* 2000; **89**: 236–241.

29. Leivonen M, Nordling S, Lundin J *et al*. p27 expression correlates with short-term, but not with long-term prognosis in breast cancer. *Breast Cancer Res Treat* 2001; **6**: 15–22.

30. Nohara T, Ryo T, Iwamoto S *et al*. Expression of cell-cycle regulator p27 is correlated to the prognosis and ER expression in breast carcinoma patients. *Oncology* 2001; **60**: 94–100.

31. Deming SL, Nass SJ, Dickson RB *et al*. C-myc amplification in breast cancer: a meta-analysis of its occurrence and prognostic relevance. *Br J Cancer* 2000; **83**: 1688–1695.

32. Mizukami Y, Nonomura A, Takizawa T *et al*. N-myc protein expression in human breast carcinoma: prognostic implications. *Anticancer Res* 1995; **15**: 2899–2905.

33. Rochlitz CF, Scott GK, Dodson JM *et al.* Incidence of activating ras oncogene mutations associated with primary and metastatic human breast cancer. *Cancer Res* 1989; **49**: 357–360.

34. Bland KI, Konstadoulakis MM, Vezeridis MP *et al.* Oncogene protein coexpression. Value of HA*ras*, c-*myc*, c-*fos*, and p53 as prognostic discriminants for breast carcinoma. *Ann Surg* 1995; **221**: 706–720.

35. Gee JM, Barroso AF, Ellis IO *et al.* Biological and clinical associations of *c-jun* activation in human breast cancer. *Int J Cancer* 2000; **89**: 177–186.

36. Liu MC, Gelmann EP. p53 gene mutations: case study of a clinical marker for solid tumors. *Semin Oncol* 2002; **29**: 246–257.

37. Gasco M, Shami S, Crook T. The p53 pathway in breast cancer. *Breast Cancer Res* 2002; **4**: 70–76.

38. Borresen-Dale AL. TP53 and breast cancer. *Hum Mutat* 2003; **21**: 292–300.

39. Bhargava V, Thor A, Deng G *et al.* The association of p53 immunopositivity with tumor proliferation and other prognostic indicators in breast cancer. *Modern Pathol* 1994; **7**: 361–368.

40. Lai H, Ma F, Trapido E, Meng L, Lai S. Spectrum of p53 tumor suppressor gene mutations and breast cancer survival. *Breast Cancer Res Treat* 2004; **83**: 57–66.

41. Rosanelli GP, Steindorfer P, Wirnsberger GH *et al.* Mutant p53 expression and DNA analysis in human breast cancer. Comparison with conventional clinicopathological parameters. *Anticancer Res* 1995; **15**: 581–586.

42. Pelosi G, Bresaola E, Rodella S *et al.* Expression of proliferating cell nuclear antigen, Ki-67 antigen, estrogen receptor protein, and tumor suppressor p53 gene in cytologic samples of breast cancer: an immunochemical study with clinical, pathobiological , and histologic correlations. *Diagn Cytopathol* 1994; **11**: 131–140.

43. Beck T, Weller EE, Weikel W *et al.* Usefulness of immunohistochemical staining for p53 in the prognosis of breast carcinomas: correlation with established prognosis parameters and with the proliferation marker, MIB-1. *Gynecol Oncol* 1995; **57**: 96–104.

44. Daidone MG, Veneroni S, Benini E *et al.* Biological markers as indicators of response to primary and adjuvant chemotherapy in breast cancer. *Int J Cancer* 1999; **84**: 580–586.

45. Kandioler-Eckersberger D, Ludwig C, Rudas M *et al.* TP53 mutation and p53 overexpression for prediction of response to neoadjuvant treatment in breast cancer patients. *Clin Cancer Res* 2000; **6**: 50–56.

46. Bertheau P, Plassa F, Espie M *et al.* Effect of mutated TP53 on response of advanced breast cancers to high-dose chemotherapy. *Lancet* 2002; **360**: 852–854.

47. Sjostrom J, Blomqvist C, Heikkila P *et al.* Predictive value of p53, mdm-2, p21, and mib-1 for chemotherapy response in advanced breast cancer. *Clin Cancer Res* 2000; **6**: 3103–3110.

48. Van Poznak C, Tan L, Panageas KS *et al.* Assessment of molecular markers of clinical sensitivity to single-agent taxane therapy for metastatic breast cancer. *J Clin Oncol* 2002; **20**: 2319–2326.

49. Hamilton A, Larsimont D, Paridaens R *et al.* A study of the value of p53, HER2, and Bcl-2 in the prediction of response to doxorubicin and paclitaxel as single agents in metastatic breast cancer: a companion study to EORTC 10923. *Clin Breast Cancer* 2000; **1**: 233–240.

50. Knoop AS, Bentzen SM, Nielsen MM *et al.* Value of epidermal growth factor receptor, HER2, p53, and steroid receptors in predicting the efficacy of tamoxifen in high-risk postmenopausal breast cancer patients. *J Clin Oncol* 2001; **19**: 3376–3384.

51. Faneyte IF, Peterse JL, Van Tinteren H *et al.* Predicting early failure after adjuvant chemotherapy in high-risk breast cancer patients with extensive lymph node involvement. *Clin Cancer Res* 2004; **10**: 4457–4463.

52. Han S, Park K, Bae BN *et al.* E2F1 expression is related with the poor survival of lymph node-positive breast cancer patients treated with fluorouracil, doxorubicin and cyclophosphamide. *Breast Cancer Res Treat* 2003; **82**: 11–16.

53. Ohene-Abuakwa Y, Pignatelli M. Adhesion molecules in cancer biology. *Adv Exp Med Biol* 2000; **465**: 115–126.

54. Skubitz AP. Adhesion molecules. *Cancer Treat Res* 2002; **107**: 305–329.

55. Beavon IR. The E-cadherin–catenin complex in tumour metastasis: structure, function

and regulation. *Eur J Cancer* 2000; **36**: 1607–1620.

56. Charpin C, Garcia S, Bonnier P *et al.* Reduced E-cadherin immunohistochemical expression in node-negative breast carcinomas correlates with 10-year survival. *Am J Clin Pathol* 1998; **109**: 431–438.

57. Parker C, Rampaul RS, Pinder SE *et al.* E-cadherin as a prognostic indicator in primary breast cancer. *Br J Cancer* 2001; **85**: 1958–1963.

58. Yoshida R, Kimura N, Harada Y *et al.* The loss of E-cadherin, alpha- and beta-catenin expression is associated with metastasis and poor prognosis in invasive breast cancer. *Int J Oncol* 2001; **18**: 513–520.

59. Gillett CE, Miles DW, Ryder K *et al.* Retention of the expression of E-cadherin and catenins is associated with shorter survival in grade III ductal carcinoma of the breast. *J Pathol* 2001; **193**: 433–441.

60. Reis-Filho JS, Cancela Paredes J, Milanezi F *et al.* Clinicopathologic implications of E-cadherin reactivity in patients with lobular carcinoma *in situ* of the breast. *Cancer* 2002; **94**: 2114–2115.

61. Chan JK, Wong CS. Loss of E-cadherin is the fundamental defect in diffuse-type gastric carcinoma and infiltrating lobular carcinoma of the breast. *Adv Anat Pathol* 2001; **8**: 165–172.

62. Kleer CG, van Golen KL, Braun T *et al.* Persistent E-cadherin expression in inflammatory breast cancer. *Modern Pathol* 2001; **14**: 458–464.

63. Burguignon LY. CD44-mediated oncogenic signaling and cytoskeleton activation during mammary tumor progression. *J Mammary Gland Biol Neoplasia* 2001; **6**: 287–297.

64. Joensuu H, Klemi PJ, Toikkanen S *et al.* Glycoprotein CD44 expression and its association with survival in breast cancer. *Am J Pathol* 1993; **143**: 866–874.

65. Guriec N, Gairard B, Marcellin L *et al.* CD44 isoforms with exon v6 and metastasis of primary N0M0 breast carcinomas. *Breast Cancer Res Treat* 1997; **44**: 261–268.

66. Schumacher U, Horny HP, Horst HA *et al.* A CD44 variant exon 6 epitope as a prognostic indicator in breast cancer. *Eur J Surg Oncol* 1996; **22**: 259–261.

67. Morris SF, O'Hanlon DM, McLaughlin R *et al.* The prognostic significance of CD44s and CD44v6 expression in stage two breast carcinoma: an immunohistochemical study. *Eur J Surg Oncol* 2001; **27**: 527–531.

68. Jansen RH, Joosten-Achjanie SR, Arends JW *et al.* CD44v6 is not a prognostic factor in primary breast cancer. *Ann Oncol* 1998; **9**: 109–111.

69. Ivaska J, Heino J. Adhesion receptors and cell invasion: mechanisms of integrin-guided degradation of extracellular matrix. *Cell Mol Life Sci* 2000; **57**: 16–24.

70. Marques LA, Franco ELF, Tortoni H *et al.* Independent prognostic value on laminin receptor expression in breast cancer survival. *Cancer Res* 1990; **50**: 1479–1483.

71. D-Errico A, Garbisa S, Liotta LA *et al.* Augmentation of type IV collagenase laminin receptor, and Ki-67 proliferation antigen associated with human colon, gastric, and breast carcinoma progression. *Modern Pathol* 1991; **4**: 239–246.

72. Daidone MG, Silvestrini R, D'Errico A *et al.* Laminin receptors, collagenase IV and prognosis in node-negative breast cancers. *Int J Cancer* 1991; **48**: 529–532.

73. Sengupta S, Chattopadhyay N, Mitra A et al. Role of alpha(v)beta3 integrin receptors in breast tumor. J Exp Clin Cancer Res. *J Exp Clin Cancer Res* 2001; **20**: 585–590.

74. Gasparini G, Brooks PC, Biganzoli E *et al.* Vascular integrin alpha(v)beta3: a new prognostic indicator in breast cancer. *Clin Cancer Res* 1998; **4**: 2625–2634.

75. Tagliabue E, Ghirelli C, Squicciarini P *et al.* Prognostic value of alpha 6 beta 4 integrin expression in breast carcinomas is affected by laminin production from tumor cells. *Clin Cancer Res* 1998; **4**: 407–410.

76. Parton M, Dowsett M, Smith I. Studies of apoptosis in breast cancer. *BMJ* 2001; **322**: 1528–1532.

77. Berardo MD, Elledge RM, de Moor C *et al.* bcl-2 and apoptosis in lymph node positive breast carcinoma. *Cancer* 1998; **82**: 1296–1302.

78. Zhang GJ, Kimijima I, Abe R *et al.* Apoptotic index correlates to bcl-2 and p53 protein expression, histological grade and prognosis in invasive breast cancers. *Anticancer Res* 1998; **18**: 1989–1998.

79. De Jong JS, van Diest PJ, Baak JP. Number of apoptotic cells as a prognostic marker in invasive breast cancer. *Br J Cancer* 2000; **82**: 368–373.

80. Gonzalez-Campora R, Galera Ruiz MR, Vazquez Ramirez F *et al*. Apoptosis in breast carcinoma. *Pathol Res Pract* 2000; **196**: 167–174.

81. Krajewski S, Krajewska M, Turner BC *et al*. Prognostic significance of apoptosis regulators in breast cancer. *Endocr Relat Cancer* 1999; **6**: 29–40.

82. Silvestrini R, Veneroni S, Daidone MG *et al*. The Bcl-2 protein: a prognostic indicator strongly related to p53 protein in lymph node-negative breast cancer patients. *J Natl Cancer Inst* 1994; **86**: 499–504.

83. McCallum M, Baker C, Gillespie K *et al*. A prognostic index for operable, node-negative breast cancer. *Br J Cancer* 2004; **90**: 1933–1941.

84. Yang Q, Sakurai T, Yoshimura G *et al*. Prognostic value of Bcl-2 in invasive breast cancer receiving chemotherapy and endocrine therapy. *Oncol Report* 2003; **10**: 121–125.

85. Sjostrom J, Blomqvist C, von Boguslawski K *et al*. The predictive value of bcl-2, bax, bcl-xL, bag-1, fas, and fasL for chemotherapy response in advanced breast cancer. *Clin Cancer Res* 2002; **8**: 811–816.

86. Vakkala M, Paakko P, Soini Y. Expression of caspases 3, 6 and 8 is increased in parallel with apoptosis and histological aggressiveness of the breast lesion. *Br J Cancer* 1999; **81**: 592–599.

87. Nakopoulou L, Alexandrou P, Stefanaki K *et al*. Immunohistochemical expression of caspase-3 as an adverse indicator of the clinical outcome in human breast cancer. *Pathobiology* 2001; **69**: 266–273.

88. Devarajan E, Sahin AA, Chen JS *et al*. Down-regulation of caspase 3 in breast cancer: a possible mechanism for chemoresistance. *Oncogene* 2002; **21**: 8843–8851.

89. Rochefort H, Chalbos D, Cunat S *et al*. Estrogen regulated proteases and antiproteases in ovarian and breast cancer cells. *J Steroid Biochem Mol Biol* 2001; **76**: 119–124.

90. Thorpe SM, Rocheford H, Garcia M et al. Association between high concentration of M52,000 cathepsin D and poor prognosis in primary breast cancer. *Cancer Res* 1989; **49**: 6008–6014.

91. Tandon AK, Clark GM, Chamness GC *et al*. Cathepsin D and prognosis in breast cancer. *N Engl J Med* 1990; **322**: 297–302.

92. Kute TE, Shao ZM, Sugg NK *et al*. Cathepsin D as a prognostic indicator for node-negative breast cancer patients using both immunoassays and enzymatic assays. *Cancer Res* 1992; **52**: 5198–5203.

93. Visscher DW, Sarkar F, LoRusso P *et al*. Immunohistologic evaluation on invasion-associated proteases in breast carcinoma. *Modern Pathol* 1993; **6**: 302–306.

94. Duffy MJ. Urokinase plasminogen activator and its inhibitor, PAI-1, as prognostic markers in breast cancer: from pilot to level 1 evidence studies. *Clin Chem* 2002; **48**: 1194–1197.

95. Harbeck N, Kates RE, Schmitt M. Clinical relevance of invasion factors urokinase-type plasminogen activator and plasminogen activator inhibitor type 1 for individualized therapy decisions in primary breast cancer is greatest when used in combination. *J Clin Oncol* 2002; **20**: 1000–1007.

96. Manders P, Tjan-Heijnen VC, Span PN *et al*. Complex of urokinase-type plasminogen activator with its type 1 inhibitor predicts poor outcome in 576 patients with lymph node-negative breast carcinoma. *Cancer* 2004; **101**: 486–494.

97. Harbeck N, Kates RE, Gauger K *et al*. Urokinase-type plasminogen activator (uPA) and its inhibitor PAI-I: novel tumor-derived factors with a high prognostic and predictive impact in breast cancer. *Thromb Haemost* 2004; **91**: 450–456.

98. Egeblad M, Werb Z. New functions for the matrix metalloproteinases in cancer progression. *Nat Rev Cancer* 2002; **2**: 161–174.

99. Brinckerhoff CE, Matrisian LM. Matrix metalloproteinases: a tail of a frog that became a prince. *Nat Rev Mol Cell Biol* 2002; **3**: 207–214.

100. McCawley LJ, Matrisian LM. Matrix metalloproteinases: multifunctional contributors to tumor progression. *Mol Med Today* 2000; **6**: 149–156.

101. Benaud C, Dickson RB, Thompson EW. Roles of the matrix metalloproteinases in mammary gland development and cancer. *Breast Cancer Res Treat* 1998; **50**: 97–116.

102. Bamias A, Dimopoulos MA. Angiogenesis in human cancer: implications in cancer therapy. *Eur J Intern Med* 2003; **14**: 459–469.

103. Dales JP, Garcia S, Carpentier S *et al*. Prediction of metastasis risk (11 year follow-up)

using VEGF-R1, VEGF-R2, Tie-2/Tek and CD105 expression in breast cancer (*n* = 905). *Br J Cancer* 2004; **90**: 1216–1221.

104. Konecny GE, Meng YG, Untch M *et al*. Association between HER-2/*neu* and vascular endothelial growth factor expression predicts clinical outcome in primary breast cancer patients. *Clin Cancer Res* 2004; **10**: 1706–1716.

105. Linderholm B, Andersson J, Lindh B *et al*. Overexpression of c-erbB-2 is related to a higher expression of vascular endothelial growth factor (VEGF) and constitutes an independent prognostic factor in primary node-positive breast cancer after adjuvant systemic treatment. *Eur J Cancer* 2004; **40**: 33–42.

106. Paik S, Shak S, Tang G *et al*. Multi-gene RT-PCR assay for predicting recurrence in node negative breast cancer patients – NSABP studies B-20 and B-14. Presented at 26th Annual San Antonio Breast Cancer Symposium. December 3–6, 2003; San Antonio, TX. Abstract #16.

107. Sorlie T, Perou CM, Tibshirani R *et al*. Gene expression patterns of breast carcinomas distinguish tumor subclasses with clinical implications. *Proc Natl Acad Sci USA* 2001; **98**: 10869–10874.

108. Bertucci F, Houlgatte R, Benziane A *et al*. Gene expression profiling of primary breast carcinomas using arrays of candidate genes. *Hum Mol Genet* 2000; **9**: 2981–2991.

109. van't Veer LJ, Dai H, van de Vijver MJ *et al*. Gene expression profiling predicts clinical outcome of breast cancer. *Nature* 2002; **415**: 530–536.

110. van de Vijver MJ, He YD, van't Veer LJ *et al*. A gene-expression signature as a predictor of survival in breast cancer. *N Engl J Med* 2002; **347**: 1999–2009.

111. Ntzani EE, Ioannidis JP. Predictive ability of DNA microarrays for cancer outcomes and correlates: an empirical assessment. *Lancet* 2003; **362**: 1439–1444.

112. Ayers M, Symmans WF, Stec J *et al*. Gene expression profiles predict complete pathologic response to neoadjuvant paclitaxel and fluorouracil, doxorubicin, and cyclophosphamide chemotherapy in breast cancer. *J Clin Oncol* 2004; **22**: 2284–2293.

113. Chang JC, Wooten EC, Tsimelzon *et al*. Gene expression profiling for the prediction of therapeutic response to docetaxel in patients with breast cancer. *Lancet* 2003; **362**: 362–369.

114. Petricoin EF, Ardekani AM, Hitt BA *et al*. Use of proteomic patterns in serum to identify ovarian cancer. *Lancet* 2002; **359**: 572–577.

115. Li J, Zhang Z, Rosenzweig J *et al*. Proteomics and bioinformatics approaches for identification of serum biomarkers to detect breast cancer. *Clin Chem* 2002; **48**: 1296–1304.

116. Paweletz CP, Trock B, Pennanen M *et al*. Proteomic patterns of nipple aspirate fluids obtained by SELDI-TOF: potential for new biomarkers to aid in the diagnosis of breast cancer. *Dis Markers* 2001; **17**: 301–307.

117. Gilbey AM, Burnett D, Coleman RE *et al*. The detection of circulating breast cancer cells in blood. *J Clin Pathol* 2004; **57**: 903–911.

118. Cristofanilli M, Budd GT, Ellis MJ *et al*. Circulating tumor cells, disease progression, and survival in metastatic breast cancer. *N Engl J Med* 2004; **351**: 781–791.

119. Szyf M, Pakneshan P, Rabbani SA. DNA methylation and breast cancer. *Biochem Pharmacol* 2004; **68**: 1187–1197.

120. Muller HM, Widschwendter A, Fiegl H *et al*. DNA methylation in serum of breast cancer patients: an independent prognostic marker. *Cancer Res* 2003; **63**: 7641–7645.

Simon S. Cross Timothy J. Stephenson
Roger D. Start

4

Digital photography in histopathology

Digital photography has enormous potential advantages for histopathologists. It provides instant display of images after capture, drastically reduces the cost of consumables, allows the simple creation of montages with labelling and annotation, and makes production of electronic presentations very simple. However, this process has produced a shift in the distribution of work away from central departments of medical illustration towards individual pathologists without any preparation or training. A survey of pathologists in the UK reveals that although 64% of them had a digital camera attached to their microscope less than 25% had received any training in digital photography.[1]

This chapter is an entirely practical account of processes in digital photography specific to histopathology written with the knowledge that we have accumulated through intensive work in this area over the past few years. We do not address the ethical issues of photography in pathology nor the use of other types of digital imaging such as videoconferencing and telepathology; for information on these, the reader is referred to other sources.[2–4]

WORKFLOW IN DIGITAL IMAGING

There is much written about the workflow in digital photography but this relates mostly to professional photographers working in fashion, sport or

Simon S. Cross MD FRCPath (for correspondence)
Reader, Academic Unit of Pathology, Division of Genomic Medicine, School of Medicine and Biomedical Sciences, University of Sheffield, Beech Hill Road, Sheffield S10 2UL, UK (E-mail: s.s.cross@sheffield.ac.uk

Timothy J. Stephenson MA MD MBA FRCPath
Consultant Histopaologist, Department of Histopathology, Royal Hallamshire Hospital, Sheffield Teaching Hospitals NHS Trust, Sheffield, UK

Roger D. Start MD FRCPath
Consultant Histopaologist, Department of Histopathology, Chesterfield Royal Hospital, Calow, Derbyshire, UK

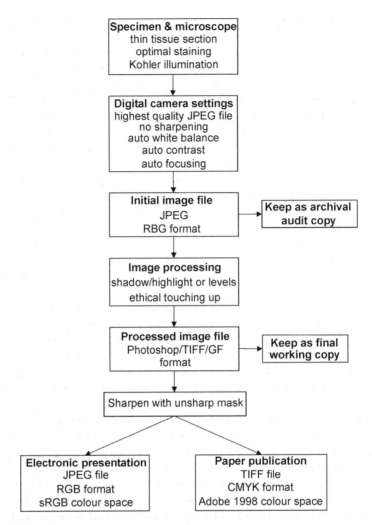

Fig. 1 Flow diagram of a recommended system of working using images captured as JPEG files in the digital camera. The different output for paper publication may be optional, more details are given in the section on submission for publication.

wildlife photography and is not relevant to histopathology.[5] Our aim is to produce high quality images for use in electronic publications or paper publications with the minimum amount of time spent processing these on a computer.

Many reference sources about digital photography suggest that, for optimal quality, an image must be captured in an uncompressed format in the camera. This should be the raw data that comes from the camera sensor (a RAW file) which can then be transformed into an image within a computer, rather than in the camera, using camera-specific software with full adjustment of colour balance and exposure before final formation of the actual image. This method requires individual processing of each image, and all image files are large requiring large memory cards in the camera, large amounts of random access memory (RAM) in the computer and a very large hard drive on which to store them. We propose an alternative workflow which is much quicker[6] and is now being recognised as entirely acceptable for professional use by well-known picture libraries.[7] The workflow is shown in Figure 1.

Images are captured and processed in the camera as Joint Photographic Expert Group (JPEG) files at the highest quality setting. These are compressed files but the compression uses a highly developed algorithm which discards only information which is virtually imperceptible to viewers. The only disadvantage of JPEG files is that the compression is recalculated every time the image is saved so if an image is stored as a JPEG file and is opened and saved several times for minor adjustments then too much information will be lost and there will be visible degradation of the image. This can be avoided by saving the initial image as an uncompressed file in Adobe Photoshop (.PSD),[8] Tagged Image File Format (.TIFF) or Genuine Fractal (.STN)[9] format whilst editing work is carried out and then converting it back to JPEG format when a final version for a specific purpose has been created.

Image processing is a relatively computer-intensive, memory-hungry process but most modern computers will have a specification adequate for this. As a minimum, we would suggest a 1 GHz processor, 256 MB of RAM and 30 GB hard drive but a 2 GHz processor, 512 MB RAM and 80 GB hard drive would produce a significant improvement in performance. We use both Windows and Macintosh operating systems and in their latest versions (Windows XP and Mac OS X) we have not found any significant differences in ease of use for digital photography. It is important to calibrate the monitor of any computer that will be used for image editing so that an edited image will appear the same on any other calibrated monitor and data projector. We have seen instances at international conferences where histological images in PowerPoint presentations have been blank white rectangles because the monitor which the speaker had used to edit images had been set at below the normal brightness setting and the data projector at the venue had been set at above normal brightness. Liquid crystal displays (LCD) are usually calibrated adequately in new computers, and probably do not need adjustment, but cathode ray tube (CRT) monitors frequently contain external controls for adjusting brightness, colour balance/temperature and contrast, and always require careful calibration. Although specialist calibrating machines and software can be purchased, the simple interactive calibration tool that accompanies Adobe Photoshop (Adobe Gamma in Windows, Monitor Calibrator in Mac OS) is effective for most purposes.

PHOTOMICROGRAPHY

CAMERA SPECIFICATION

The main specification of digital cameras which is used in marketing and superficial comparisons is the total number of pixels in the camera sensor (the digital 'film' equivalent). This is usually given as 'megapixels' which equates to millions of pixel elements. Thus a 3-megapixel camera will contain about 3 million pixel elements and produce an image size of 2048 x 1536 pixels in 4:3 ratio format. The number of megapixels that are required is dependent on the purpose of the images. Clearly, an image which is 2048 x 1536 pixels will be in excess of that required in an electronic presentation since most data projectors display an image at a resolution of 1024 x 768 pixels. When publishing images in print there is a greater demand for higher resolution. Publishers usually stipulate that images are reproduced at 300 lines per inch, which is equivalent to 300 pixels per inch. Thus a 3 megapixel image would give a printed image of 6.8 x 5 inches at 300 pixels per inch – this fills half a page of A4 paper which is adequate for any illustrations in books and research papers. If larger images are required for printed publications, then either a camera with more pixel elements is needed or software which interpolates pixels between existing pixels to upsize an image should be used (see integration into posters section below). For most purposes in histopathology, a 3-megapixel camera is adequate but in the consumer market 5 megapixels seems to be the new standard and this would give sufficient resolution for full A4-size printed images. One caution with cameras with large numbers of megapixels is that generally the size of the sensor remains the same so each pixel element is smaller. Thus, in an 8-megapixel camera each pixel element may be less than half the size of that in a 3-megapixel element. This means that each pixel element will receive a smaller number of photons for the same exposure and so the sensitivity of the pixels has to be higher in a camera with more megapixels for the same light level. This leads to increased problems with electronic noise caused by inappropriate signals from pixel elements. This is the reason that professional photographers use digital cameras with larger sensors and correspondingly larger pixel elements, and would use a 6 megapixel digital single lens reflex camera in preference to an 8 megapixel compact digital camera.

The aspect ratio of the camera sensor is also a consideration. Most consumer digital cameras have an aspect ratio of 4:3 (ratio of image width to height) which is very convenient for electronic presentations since it is the same ratio as computer monitor screens and data projectors. Single lens reflex digital cameras mostly retain the aspect ratio of 35-mm film which is 3:2 and so will leave areas of space on the computer screen at the top and bottom when displayed at full width. The 3:2 ratio was only derived from a mechanical constraint in the first 35-mm film cameras and the 4:3 ratio is much more useful in most contexts.

OTHER FEATURES

Digital cameras for photomicroscopy will obviously have to connect to an existing microscope. Specialised cameras are available from microscope manufacturers which are specifically designed for individual microscopes. These generally work very well but the cost is usually much higher than the more common solution of attaching a consumer digital camera to a microscope via a special relay lens. This relay lens is attached by the filter screw at the front of the camera lens so any digital camera under consideration must have this feature and an appropriate relay lens must be available.

Some thought needs to be given to how images will be monitored during photography. All digital cameras have LCD monitor screens to view images before and after they have been captured and this can be used to compose photomicrographs. However, unless the camera has a twist-and-tilt body/LCD screen, then that screen will be at the top of the microscope facing the ceiling which is very inconvenient. Most digital cameras have a video output so it is possible to connect them to a video monitor situated next to the microscope and view images on this. Since the autofocus function on most digital cameras produces well-focused images the monitor screen only needs to be used for image composition and so a twist-and-tilt LCD monitor facing the user on top of the microscope is a convenient and space-saving mode of monitoring. Consumer digital cameras have four barriers to taking photographs which are very irritating to those used to quality film cameras:

- *they take at least a few seconds to become active after switching on*

- *there is an appreciable pause between depressing the shutter button and actual capture of the image*

- *images cannot be captured in rapid succession*

- *the battery life is very short especially if images are viewed on the LCD screen.*

Since photomicroscopy does not have the same time pressures as sports photography, the shutter release lag is unimportant: the start-up time and battery life are easily circumvented by use of a mains adaptor allowing the camera to be left permanently on. A mechanical or electronic remote shutter release is usually required to prevent camera and microscope shake at the relatively low shutter speeds that are often needed.

CAMERA SET-UP

All digital cameras contain a plethora of features which need to be set correctly, or disabled, when taking photomicrographs. We have found that most functions work very well when left in their automatic mode. These include focusing, contrast, and white balance. The only time that we do not use automatic white balance is when we are taking a sequence of photographs which will make up a montage, *e.g.* serial sections with different immunohistochemical stains. In such a series, the background needs to appear identical in all the images. To achieve this, we set up the camera and illumination to produce the optimal image and then move the slide on the stage to a blank area with no tissue but which is still under the coverslip. We then use the camera menu to set the white balance to this preset value and take all the pictures using this white balance, without changing the illumination or any other microscope settings. We disable any in-camera sharpening and use a sharpening filter in an image editing program (see below).

TRANSFER OF IMAGES TO A COMPUTER

There are two common methods of transferring images from a digital camera to a computer: (i) direct transfer from the camera to the computer via a USB or Firewire interface; or (ii) removal of the memory card from the camera and transfer of its contents to a computer via a card reader. The latter method has the advantage that it is generally quicker and means that the computer does not have to be adjacent to the camera. The two main operating systems on computers, Windows XP and Macintosh OS X, both contain excellent intrinsic systems for importing and showing images. These operating systems will usually recognise any card reader that is plugged into a USB or Firewire interface without additional software, and will automatically activate a self-explanatory importing programme when a memory card is plugged into such a reader. We would caution against installing any software that is included with the digital camera (with the exception of a well-known image editing programme, such as Adobe Photoshop Elements or Paintshop Pro) since this is unnecessary and is likely to install itself as the default application for all images, making transfer and editing of images difficult with any other program.

MACRO PHOTOGRAPHY

Macroscopic photography in pathology has no special differences from any other type of macro photography; general photography books which cover this area will be useful for pathologists.[10,11] The ideal equipment for macro photography would be a digital, single-lens reflex camera with a dedicated macro lens and the cost of such a set up is falling all the time (currently about £1100 for a 6-megapixel digital SLR with a 90-mm macro lens). Such equipment would give professional quality images that could be used in any type of publication. However, satisfactory macro images can be made using a standard consumer digital camera. Most of these cameras have a macro setting which allows close focusing; if this is not sufficient to display the intended feature, then many have an inexpensive close-up lens which can be screwed to the filter thread in front of the lens.

Lighting of the specimen is the key to successful macro photography and it well worth investing in a dedicated lighting system which can be used in the cut-up area.[12] A great advantage of digital cameras is that they have many different preprogramed and automatic white balance mechanisms which allows a wide variety of lighting sources. With film cameras a specific film would have to be used for tungsten lighting or coloured filters to correct the green cast from fluorescent lighting. The white balance function on digital cameras means that almost any lighting source will be suitable. Colour balance problems may arise when a specimen is lit by two different types of light source, such as tungsten and fluorescent, and an overall white balance correction will not be able to produce a satisfactory correction. For this reason, it is best to use light from only one type of source (e.g. tungsten), and to avoid areas where there is a strong, but not exclusive, lighting contribution from daylight.

Since digital cameras can correct for most lighting colour casts, it is possible to use sources which would not have been considered for film cameras. The most useful of these are small fluorescent sources which do not generate heat and thus have a great advantage over tungsten illumination since they will not cause an increase in fumes from formalin-fixed specimens.[12] Specialist companies produce useful fluorescent light sources and diffusing boxes into which specimens could be placed for macro photography (e.g. Bowens Trilite and Cocoon).[13] It should be noted that non-specialist fluorescent light sources may have strobe-like fluctuations in intensity at a rate that may affect the exposure calculations of the camera, producing apparently random fluctuations of over- or under-exposure. Although most digital cameras have dedicated white balance settings for tungsten and fluorescent lighting, the automatic white balance setting is generally ideal for most macro photography. In most macro photography, the aim will be to display the whole photographed area in sharp focus which will require a small lens aperture and a correspondingly slow shutter speed, so most macro set-ups will require a solid mounting for the camera, *i.e.* a heavy tripod or a dedicated overhead camera stand and a remote shutter release to avoid any blurring from camera shake.

PROCESSING DIGITAL IMAGES

COLOUR BALANCE AND SHADOW/HIGHLIGHT ADJUSTMENT

Although we take great care in setting up the microscope and camera when taking digital photomicrographs, we still find that all images require a small amount of editing to make them appear bright and crisp. This contrasts with digital photographs of scenery and people in sunny weather which can usually be displayed without any editing straight from the camera. The reason for this appears to be that photomicrographs present unusual images, often with large areas of white in the background of lower power or small biopsy images and a very restricted colour spectrum due to the haematoxylin and eosin or immunohistochemical staining. We have experimented extensively with all the different colour balance settings on digital cameras, the microscope illumination and all combinations of aperture/shutter speed/manual exposure settings but have still not managed to produce images which do not require a small amount of editing.

There are a number of image-editing programs available but the industry standard is Adobe Photoshop.[8] Paintshop Pro[14] is a lower cost alternative product which provides many functions that are similar to Photoshop. Photoshop is produced in a number of different versions with differing levels of complexity. Many digital cameras are supplied with a complimentary copy of Photoshop LE which contains all the basic functions including the important 'Unsharp Mask' function. Photoshop Elements is a more feature-rich version which is designed for the average consumer digital photographer and a new version of this (Photoshop Elements 3) contains many extra useful features. The full version of Photoshop, currently named Photoshop CS2 (equivalent to version 9), is expensive even with an educational discount but does contain a number of features which we use all the time to process images and which are not currently available in other versions.

The most important of these are the 'Shadow/Highlight' tool, the 'Lab Color' mode and the 'Healing Brush' tool. We have found that a single adjustment using the 'Shadow/Highlight' tool produces a dramatic brightening of images with a crisp white background which is superior to other methods using the 'Levels' tool. In this method, we open the image in Photoshop, select the 'Shadow/Highlight' tool from the 'Image-Adjustments' menu and enter 1% into the amount box at the top of the dialogue box (it is set to 50% by default) and click 'OK'. This is the only adjustment that we have found necessary for the vast majority of images before they are sharpened. Since this amount is always 1%, it can be incorporated into an automated

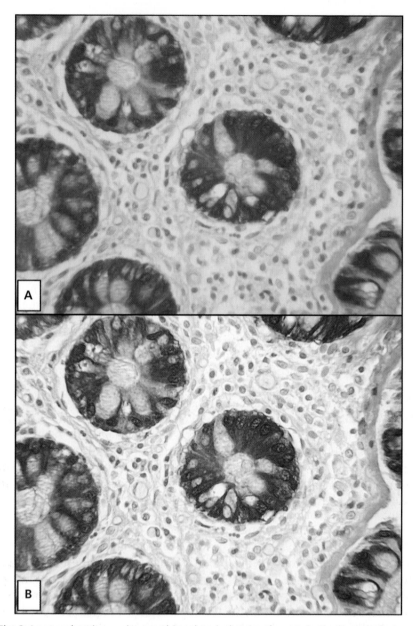

Fig. 2 Images showing an immunohistochemical stain of crypts in the large bowel before (a) and after (b) image processing. The only processing that was applied to the image was to lift the shadows by 1% using the 'Shadow/Highlight' tool and then sharpening using the 'Unsharp Mask' filter. The process was automated as a Photoshop 'Action' shown in Figure 3, and took one click and 6 s to perform.

Photoshop Action and an image can be fully processed by clicking a single button (Figs 2 and 3). Our Photoshop Actions carrying out these processes for the haematoxylin and eosin stain, cytological preparations and immunohistochemical stains are freely downloadable from the Web.[15] The 'Healing Brush' tool is ideal for removing unwanted artefacts in the image

Action: H&E ×10 lens
     Shadow/Highlight
          Shadow: Parameters
          Amount: 1%
          Tone Width: 50%
          Radius: 30
          Highlight: Parameters
          Amount: 0%
          Tone Width: 50%
          Radius: 30
          Black Clip: 0.01
          White Clip: 0.01
          Contrast: 0
          Color Correction: 20
     Convert Mode
          To: Lab color mode
     Select lightness channel
     Unsharp Mask
          Amount: 150%
          Radius: 3 pixels
          Threshold: 0
     Convert Mode
          To: RGB color mode

Fig. 3 The Photoshop Action that was used to process the image shown in Figure 2. Note that this Action was simply recorded within Photoshop without the need to type all these parameters into a text file. The full set of Actions that we have developed is freely available for downloading from the Web.[15]

such as dust particles but of course must only be used for image optimisation and not unethical image manipulation.[2] The 'Lab Color' mode is used in advanced sharpening techniques (see below).

SHARPENING

The majority of digital cameras have an anti-aliasing filter in front of the sensor which causes minor blurring of the image (which is its purpose so that strange aberrations do not appear when objects with small regular patterns are photographed). This means that all digital photographs require sharpening at some stage before final output. Digital cameras all have sharpening routines built into them and the default setting for the camera is usually to have some in-camera sharpening of the image. For many purposes, such as electronic presentation of macroscopic images (*e.g.* colorectal cancer resections), this is useful because it means that images can be transferred straight from the camera into the presentation without any intermediary step. However, if the image may be used for any other purpose, such as publication in print, then the in-camera sharpening must be switched off and a sharpening filter applied at the end of any image processing and resizing work on the image.

Practical experience also shows that photomicroscopic images require a higher level of sharpening than macroscopic images and this is more easily

Table 1 Suggested values for user-specified parameters when using the 'Unsharp Mask' filter

Objective lens on microscope	Amount	Radius in pixels	Threshold in pixels
Macroscopic	80–120%	1	4
x2.5	100–200%	2	0
x4	100–200%	2.5	0
x10	100–200%	3	0
x20	100–200%	4	0
x40	100–200%	4.5	0

controlled in an image-editing program than within the digital camera. Image-editing software often offers a range of sharpening filters including sharpen, sharpen edges, sharpen more and unsharp mask. The latter, counter-intuitively named, filter is the most powerful sharpening tool which is used by all professional digital photographers. This filter has three adjustable parameters – amount, radius and threshold. We have found that the values for these which produce the best results for photomicrographs are very different from those recommended for photographs of people and landscapes. We set the amount at 100–200%, the threshold to zero and the radius at a value that varies with the magnification of the objective lens, our suggested values are given in Table 1. At higher values of radius, this filter introduces significant amounts of noise so the minimal value required to give an adequately sharp image should be used. It is interesting that it is only the black and white component of the image that requires sharpening to give the overall visual effect of sharpening. This can be used to advantage if image quality is paramount since the black and white components can be sharpened separately using a function such as the lightness channel in the 'Lab Color' mode of Adobe Photoshop and then the colour components returned to produce a sharp image with much lower levels of noise.[16]

Sharpening should be applied to an image only after all other desired functions have been performed, including resizing of the image, otherwise its effect will be diminished. Some publishers ask for unsharpened images which they sharpen at the page layout stage. Images in electronic presentations, especially heavily compressed images on web pages, require a much higher degree of sharpening to produce an adequately sharp effect with quite extreme values for radius and amount.[16]

INTEGRATION INTO ELECTRONIC PRESENTATIONS

It is very easy to integrate digital images into electronic presentations. The Windows XP and Mac OS X operating systems have slide-show functions which are a very simple way of showing images on a monitor screen or data projector, and would be the most time- efficient system of showing images at a multidisciplinary team meeting (*e.g.* macroscopic images of colorectal cancer resections). However, most histopathology presentations will need to include some text and some labelling of images and the vast majority of histopathologists use the Microsoft PowerPoint programme to do this.[17] Images can be imported singly into PowerPoint slides using the 'Insert → Picture → From File' function. If a large number of images are to be included in a PowerPoint presentation, then it is much quicker to use the 'Insert → Picture → New Photo Album' function which enables a user to insert any number of pictures selected from the internal hard drive or external connected sources and automatically scales each image to fill a single slide. It is easier to use this function as the basis for a new presentation since it creates a new, separate file rather than adds images to an existing presentation, but slides can be easily moved between presentations using 'Copy and Paste' functions.

Images can be easily resized within the PowerPoint programme by dragging corner markers or by double-clicking on the image and entering absolute size measurements into the height and width boxes. It is much easier to add any text, labelling and arrows to images within the PowerPoint program since these will remain as individually editable elements which can be changed at will and copied between slides to provide continuity of presentation style. If text and labelling is added to an image in an image-editing program, such as Adobe Photoshop, then it will be embedded within the image file when saved to a format suitable for importing into PowerPoint and no further editing can be made within PowerPoint itself.

Size of image file is an important consideration when using a large number of digital images in a PowerPoint presentation. If there are many large image files in a presentation then the total size of the presentation can amount to many megabytes, often over a hundred. This file size is an underestimate of the total amount of RAM required to display it, since the embedded images are usually JPEG files that will require decompression to display them. If such a presentation is being shown on a computer that has a relatively small amount RAM (*e.g.* 128 MB), then the size of the presentation, the operating system and PowerPoint program will exceed the amount of available RAM. When this occurs two things may happen: (i) the computer will not display any further images in the presentation replacing them with a large red cross; or (ii) the computer will have to transfer components between the RAM and the hard drive (buffering) which may cause long delays in the transition between slides. If you are using your own laptop computer to make a presentation, then you will find this out before you use it in earnest (assuming you run through the presentation beforehand); however, at many conference venues, presentations have to be loaded onto a computer within the lecture theatre or onto a central server and you will not know how much RAM this computer will have.

It is thus prudent to reduce the size of a PowerPoint presentation so that it will run successfully in the minimum amount of RAM that could be reasonably expected to be present in a venue computer (currently 128 MB so keep the presentation size below 50 MB). It is very easy to reduce the size of images in a presentation without any compromise in the quality of image that will be presented through a data projector. The size of file can be reduced by resizing the image to the same pixel resolution as the data projector or by compressing the JPEG file more heavily, or a combination of the two. The current most frequent resolution of data projectors is 1024 x 768 pixels (XGA) though this is likely to continue to rise over the next few years with UXGA

(1600 x 1200 pixels), the next higher standard. If an image from a 3-megapixel camera is reduced from its native 2048 x 1536 pixel size to 1024 x 768 pixels, then its uncompressed size will fall from 9.2 MB to 2.25 MB. JPEG compression is also very effective at reducing file size with no apparent change in image quality.

We have experimented with various compression ratios using blind side-by-side comparisons of images and it is possible to compress a 9.2 MB image from a 3-megapixel camera down to 80 KB (0.08 MB) with no perceived loss of quality in an electronic presentation. With these levels of compression, a 100-image presentation – the sort of size that is often needed for a slide seminar – could be contained in a total file size of 10 MB which would run on any reasonably modern computer. It would be very time consuming to open and resave 100 images individually at a higher JPEG compression ratio but fortunately this can be done automatically using a batch processing function in any common image editing programme such as Adobe Photoshop or Paintshop Pro. The single batch processing event could contain a number of different functions including resizing the image, converting it to sRGB colour space (if it was in a different colour space), sharpening of the images to a level suitable for an electronic publication and saving it at a higher JPEG compression ratio.

INTEGRATION INTO POSTERS

Putting digital images into posters is a very similar process to inserting them into electronic publications. Most conference presenters now produce their posters on a single large sheet of paper using design software and printed out on wide format inkjet printers. Although there would be some significant advantages to using software specifically designed for producing printed output, such as Quark Xpress or Adobe InDesign, many pathologists produce their own posters. However, the learning curve for such software is too steep to justify its use a few times a year. Thus, most pathologists use PowerPoint to produce posters; the procedures are largely the same as creating electronic presentations.

The only aspect which may require additional work concerns the size of the images as they will appear on the final printed poster. The usual specified resolution of printed images is 300 dots per inch so an image from a 3-megapixel camera can be printed to a maximum size of 6.8 x 5 inches before there is possible image degradation. In practice, the image can been printed at a slightly larger size without visible artefact but if it is to be printed at a much larger size then some form of image upsizing is needed. The general principle of upsizing software is to interpolate pixels between existing pixels to make the image larger but without significant degradation. The process examines the pixels around the potential interpolation space and uses an algorithm to determine the best choice of pixel. If the space is in the middle of a homogeneous patch of colour, then the decision is simple: put an identical pixel in the space. If the space is in an area of high detail or the boundary between two different coloured areas, then the decision is more difficult. There are now several sophisticated software packages which can upsize images with virtually no visible degradation – Shortcut PhotoZoom Pro (S-Spline)[18] and Genuine Fractals[9] are the two best known. Using these programs, it is possible to upsize a 6-megapixel image to a size that will fill the side of a double-decker bus. It should be noted that the base level of information in an image is important and there is an important practical threshold between about 3 and 6 megapixel images with those of 6 megapixels and above producing much better quality upsized images. However, if the upsizing required is only moderate, then the 'Image Size' function from the 'Image' menu within Adobe Photoshop can be used as an iterative process in 10% increments to produce very acceptable image quality.[19]

SUBMISSION FOR PUBLICATION

Most publishers now require images to be submitted in electronic format even if they still ask for hard copy whilst a manuscript is reviewed and edited. Publishers give specific instructions about the format of images and these need to be noted, but there are some common features. The major consideration for publishable images is whether they are of sufficient resolution to produce a high quality image at the size at which they will be printed. This can be calculated by taking the pixel dimensions of the image, say 2048 x 1536 pixels, and divide by 300 to give the size in inches, since the printing density is usually 300 dots per inch. We have shown in the section on camera specification that a 3-megapixel camera will produce a printed image which is 6.8 x 5 inches, sufficient for half-page illustrations on A4 pages. When we take digital images and view them on a computer screen, we are using an image that is basically coded in three colour components (red, green and blue – RGB). When a publisher prints an image on a commercial printing press they will be using a four colour printing process (cyan, magenta, yellow and key – CMYK). When we view an image on screen, it will generally be displayed using the colour space of the computer monitor which will be sRGB whereas a commercial printing process can display a wider range of darkness and lightness for each colour that is present in the Adobe 1998 colour space. Thus, at some point between image capture and commercial printing, there has to be a conversion of the image format from an RGB format in sRGB colour space to a CMYK format in Adobe 1998 colour space.

Many publishers state that the submission format should be an uncompressed TIFF file in CMYK format and Adobe 1998 colour space and this may cause some problems for the submitting pathologist since some image-editing software will not support this conversion. The full version of Adobe Photoshop will perform this conversion but the LE version that is often included as free software with a digital camera, and Adobe Photoshop Elements, do not. Does this mean that all pathologists who submit images for publications need to buy the expensive full version of Photoshop or a similar image editing program? We would suggest that this is unnecessary since the publishers will always have a huge range of software that will perform such conversions, and their image editing staff are likely to be more skilled at this than submitting pathologists. In reality, it appears that the essential factor is the image quality and any other formatting issues can be dealt with by the publishers.

We all work closely with publishers in a number of roles and we generally submit images as JPEG files saved at the highest quality (*i.e.* lowest compression ratio), in RGB format and sRGB colour space and we have never had any images returned for reformatting. If a figure has been produced in PowerPoint because labelling and annotations had to be added, then this can generally be submitted as a PowerPoint file and again the publishers will be able to carry out the necessary conversion. A problem that we have encountered recently with PowerPoint files is when submission of manuscripts is entirely electronic and it is stipulated (and indeed the web site will only accept) the figures must be JPEG files (presumably so that the files are smaller and thus easier to distribute electronically for refereeing). It is possible to save a PowerPoint presentation as a JPEG file using the 'Save As' function from the 'File' menu within PowerPoint; however, it does not appear possible to adjust the compression ratio for this process and the default values produce an extremely compressed image of poor quality. We have found a solution to this which requires the use of the full version of Adobe Acrobat[8] (rather than the Adobe Acrobat Reader program that is pre-installed on most new computers). With this program, it is possible to convert a PowerPoint presentation into a high quality Portable Document File (PDF) which can then itself be converted to a high quality JPEG file within the Acrobat program.

PRINTING

Many journals have moved to completely electronic submission so the need to print out images has markedly decreased. In many cases, the first time that an image is printed onto paper is the page proof of a book or journal. However, there is still some need to print images for journals that still have paper submission and for local production of teaching materials. The main aim, and problem, with printing digital images is to produce a printed version that has the same appearances as on the computer screen. The most effective way of doing this is to have a reasonable system of colour management that flows from the capture of the image through to the final printing of the image. Professional imaging companies who produce printed images will take images of standardised colour targets in any run of images which can then be used to adjust colour balance in an image-editing program on computers with carefully calibrated monitors. These images will then be directed to a printer which has also been calibrated to produce a colour management profile which accurately reflects the on-screen appearances.[20] Such companies will also ensure that all their computer screens are set up in constant ambient lighting conditions of a known colour temperature and that all prints are examined in a similarly controlled lighting environment.

None of these conditions will be available to most pathologists but there are a number of simple steps that can be taken to produce consistent and high-quality printed output. The computer monitor must be calibrated (see section on computer specification above) and it is best to view the screen in low ambient lighting conditions avoiding bright sunlight falling on the screen or close to it. Change the background of your image- editing program (and your computer 'desktop' screen if this is visible) to a neutral grey colour to avoid bright colours adjacent to the image from altering your perception of the image colours. Inkjet colour printers are the most appropriate output device since they offer high resolution with a blending of individual ink droplets on the paper which produces a smooth image similar to conventional photographs.[21] Colour laser printers are not appropriate for photographic images since the resolution is lower and the particles of toner do not blend together producing an apparently 'pixelated' image even from very high quality electronic images. Such printers are actually designed for high volume output of documents with blocks of homogeneous colour such as letterheads and brochures with graphic, rather than photographic, images.

The technology of inkjet printers has advanced so rapidly that virtually any inkjet printer costing over £80 will produce excellent publication-quality images. The main manufacturers are Hewlett-Packard, Canon and Epson, with professional photographers appearing to favour the latter; this is probably due to their early development of archival inks and fine art quality papers rather than any other significant difference from other manufacturers. The main expense of using inkjet printers is the print cartridges which are now so complex that they constitute the entire printing head rather than just a reservoir of printing ink. Each manufacturer has developed their ink cartridges and printing papers as a combination to produce the best possible quality. Although this means that they tie the user into their expensive consumables (and as a result they can sell their printers as loss leaders), this does seem to produce the best results; much less satisfactory prints will be produced using cheaper generic inks and paper.

For photographic output, the expensive glossy coated 'photo quality' papers have to be used as ordinary paper is much too absorbent to produce well-defined images with the desired colour balance. It is possible to use ordinary paper as a draft output to check that the image appears at the desired size in the desired position on the page, but no assessment of image quality or colour balance should be made until it has been printed on the final output glossy photographic paper as any corrections to colour balance based on the draft output will be erroneous.

Most printers come with quite extensive software which can again appear to 'take over' the computer on which they are installed – to the extent of prompting the user to order new ink cartridges from a specific source on the web when levels are running low. As with the software that accompanies digital cameras, it is best to install the bare minimum of software that will operate the printer. It is often possible to download a 'business' driver for a specific printer from the manufacturer's website which will provide just the bare driver without any other computer-clogging 'consumer' software. It is best to print an image using software that contains sensible colour management software that will provide an optimal interface with the printer. Printing from within an image-editing program, such as Adobe Photoshop, can provide very consistent colour management with no further effort from the user. We have had very successful results using the 'Print With Preview' function available on the 'File' menu in Photoshop. In the dialogue box that appears with this function, we select 'Document' colour space in the 'Source Space' option and 'Printer Color Management' in the 'Printer Space' option. PowerPoint is not generally a good program to use to print images since its colour management is not as consistent as an image-editing program. An

Table 2 Properties and costs of storage options

Device	Maximum storage capacity	Interface with computer	Cost	Cost per MB of storage	Permanence	Suggested uses
Zip drive	750 MB	Zip drive through USB or Firewire	£90 for drive, £9 per disc	1p	Volatile magneto-optical	Transfer of images and presentations between computers
Memory cards	4 GB	Card reader through USB or Firewire	£75 for 1 GB	7.5p	Volatile solid state – not susceptible to X-rays but susceptible to electromagnetic forces	Recording images in digital camera
Data pens	4 GB	USB	£90 for 1 GB	9p	Volatile solid state – not susceptible to X-rays but susceptible to electromagnetic forces	Transfer of images and presentations between computers
Recordable compact disc (CDR)	750 MB	CDR drive	£0.11 per disc	0.01p	Semi-permanent, susceptible to strong sunlight	Transfer of images and presentations between computers, archiving of images
Recordable digital versatile disc (DVD)	4 GB	DVD drive	£0.48 per disc	0.01p	Semi-permanent, susceptible to strong sunlight	Transfer of images and presentations between computers, archiving of images
External hard drive	250 GB or more	USB or Firewire	£160 for 250 GB	0.06p	Volatile magnetic	Easily accessible archive of images which is too large to remain on computer's internal hard drive

Costs in UK£ or pence (p).

alternative method of printing images is to send them to a company that will print them on to high quality photographic paper using a three-colour laser. This has the advantage of producing archival quality images that will not fade for many years and the cost per print may be slightly cheaper than the cost of ink and paper on an inkjet printer. Such services are becoming more available at conventional photographic processing shops but can also be accessed by the internet.[22]

STORAGE AND INDEXING

The instant results and absence of consumable costs in digital photography mean that most users take many more images than they would have done with film-based photography. This leads to a need for large storage capacity and effective indexing of images. The different storage options are summarised in Table 2. We have found that portable external hard drives are the best devices for storing large archives of images to which we require access but which either exceed the capacity of the internal hard drive of our main computer or to which we need access from more than one computer. External hard drives are magnetic storage media which cannot be considered to be permanent so batch archiving onto recordable CDs or DVDs should be employed as secure method of backup. USB data pens are a rapid and re-usable method of transferring images and presentations between computers but are again a volatile form of storage, which are sensitive to electromagnetic forces such as airport metal detectors; for important presentations at conferences, it is best to create a copy on a CD.

When 35-mm film slides were the main method of presentation, pathologists stored their slides in plastic display wallets in filing cabinets. The wallets might have contained a whole lecture or a set of slides on a particular theme (*e.g.* endometrial pathology). The wallets may have had protruding tabs onto which labels were attached so a particular sheet could be identified easily. This system appeared to work very effectively for most pathologists. An entirely analogous system can be created within the Windows and Macintosh operating systems with electronic folders labelled with particular themes and the view option set to display thumbnails of each image. Such a system has virtually no set-up time and will work very effectively with careful labelling. The electronic storage of images does give great potential for indexing systems based on keywords attached to each image file and it would be possible to set up a system where all available images could be searched by simple text searches (*e.g.* 'endometrium' and 'cancer'). However, such systems require a lot of input from the user and are unlikely to repay this time if only a single user is storing and retrieving images. These systems would be very helpful for indexing departmental collections of images with appropriate resources for the indexing process. One advantage of these image management systems is that they will search all storage devices on a computer for all types of images and display these in one large catalogue file so images cannot be 'lost' in obscure folders in unlikely parts of the filing system. Two programs which are popular for image management are Adobe Photoalbum[8] and iView Media Pro,[23] with the latter being the most frequent choice amongst professional photographers.

Points for best practice

- Highest quality JPEG files are the format of choice for image capture in digital cameras.

- Uncompressed Photoshop or TIFF files are the format of choice for archived and working copies of digital images.

- JPEG files at appropriate compression ratios in RGB colour mode are the format of choice for electronic presentations.

- TIFF files in CMYK colour mode are the format of choice for submissions for paper publication.

- Recordable CDs or DVDs are the most appropriate semi-permanent archival storage media.

- External hard drives are the best storage medium for collections of images that exceed the capacity of the native internal hard drive.

ACKNOWLEDGEMENTS

We are grateful for the financial assistance of the medical charities NEDSCAN and Nursing a Dream for funding our work in digital imaging.

References

1. Dennis T, Start RD, Cross SS. The use of digital imaging, video conferencing and telepathology in histopathology: a national survey. *J Clin Pathol* 2005; **58**: 254–258.
2. Tranberg HA, Rous BA, Rashbass J. Legal and ethical issues in the use of anonymous images in pathology teaching and research. *Histopathology* 2003; **42**: 104–109.
3. Bamford WM, Rogers N, Kassam M, Rashbass J, Furness PN. The development and evaluation of the UK national telepathology network. *Histopathology* 2003; **42**: 110–119.
4. Cross SS, Dennis T, Start RD. Telepathology: current status and future prospects in diagnostic histopathology. *Histopathology* 2002; **41**: 1–19.
5. Rouse A. *Digital SLR Masterclass*. Lewes: Photographers' Institute Press, 2004.
6. Rockwell K. JPG vs RAW vs TIFF: *Get it Right the First Time* <http://www.kenrockwell.com/tech/raw.htm>.
7. Alamy Stock Photography <http://www.alamy.com>.
8. Adobe Systems Inc., San Jose, CA <http://www.adobe.com/>.
9. Genuine Fractals. LizardTech Inc., Seattle, WA <http://www.lizardtech.com/>.
10. Freeman M. *Close-up Photography: The Definitive Guide for Serious Digital Photographers*. Lewes: Ilex, 2004.
11. Harcourt Davis P. *Small Things Big: Close-up and Macro Photography*. London: David & Charles, Quarto Publishing plc, 2003.
12. Freeman M. *Light and Lighting: The Definitive Guide for Serious Digital Photographers*. Lewes: Ilex, 2004.
13. Bowens International, Clacton on Sea <http://www.bowens.co.uk/>.
14. Paint Shop Pro, JASC Software, Purley <http://www.jasc.com/en/?>.
15. Cross SS. *Photoshop Actions for Processing Photomicrographs* <http://www.pathcentral.org.uk/photoshop.htm>.
16. Kelby S. Lab color sharpening. In: Kelby S. (ed) *The Photoshop Book for Digital Photographers*. Indianapolis, IN: New Riders Publishing, 2003; 298–304.

17. PowerPoint, Microsoft Corporation, Seattle, WA <http://www.microsoft.com/>.

18. Shortcut PhotoZoom Pro (S-Spline), Shortcut Software Development BV, The Netherlands <http://www.trulyphotomagic.com/>

19. Kelby S. Resizing digital camera photos. In: Kelby S. (ed) *The Photoshop Book for Digital Photographers*. Indianapolis, IN: New Riders Publishing, 2003; 64–66.

20. Fraser B. *Real World Color Management: Industrial-Strength Production Techniques*. Berkeley, CA: Peachpit, 2004.

21. Johnson H. *Mastering Digital Printing: The Photographer's and Artist's Guide to High-Quality Digital Output*. Cincinnati, OH: Muska & Lipman, 2003.

22. Colormailer, Colorplaza Ltd, Vevey, Switzerland <http://www.colormailer.com/>.

23. iView Media Pro, iView Multimedia Ltd, London <http://www.iview-multimedia.com/>.

Cyril Fisher

5

Gastrointestinal stromal tumours

Gastrointestinal stromal tumours (GISTs) are mesenchymal tumours arising in the gastrointestinal tract and occasionally elsewhere within the abdomen. The earlier literature classified them as smooth muscle or nerve sheath tumours but, even in the benign examples, evidence for such differentiation was difficult to find. Mazur and Clark introduced the term stromal tumour in 1983[1] after they failed to find ultrastructural evidence of smooth muscle or nerve sheath differentiation in several gastric tumours. Neoplasms showing only these types of differentiation now comprise fewer than 20% of gastrointestinal mesenchymal tumours and, like those of fibroblastic or vascular type, are conventionally excluded from the definition of GIST.

GISTs have recently undergone a conceptual revolution, with the hypothesis that many of them show differentiation towards (and supposedly arise from a precursor of) interstitial cells of Cajal which are normally concerned with motility of the gut. This category is considered to subsume the ultrastructurally-defined rare lesions previously known as gastrointestinal autonomic nerve tumours (GANTs).[2] The availability of specific antibodies and clarification of the immunohistochemical profile of GISTs have facilitated their diagnosis. However, careful morphological examination and clinicopathological correlation remain essential for excluding mimics and for predicting behaviour in this group of neoplasms.

INCIDENCE AND DISTRIBUTION

GISTs comprise 5–20% of all sarcomas (for comparison, 15% of sarcomas arise in retroperitoneum and 42% in extremities), and represent about 1% of all gastrointestinal malignancies. Malignant GISTs are rare with an incidence of

Cyril Fisher MA MD DSc FRCPath
Professor of Tumour Pathology, Department of Histopathology, Royal Marsden Hospital, Fulham Road, London SW3 6JJ, UK (E-mail: cyril.fisher@rmh.nhs.uk)

about 5 per million of population (compared with 25 per million for soft tissue sarcomas). They are most common in adults aged 50–60 years, and vary in prognosis according to their location within the gastrointestinal tract. About 5% of GISTs are oesophageal, 50–70% involve the stomach, 25–40% the small intestine (of which 10–20% arise in duodenum, 27–37% in jejunum, 27–53% in ileum) and fewer than 10% are colorectal (50% colonic, 50% rectal).[3] GIST-type tumours arising in omentum, peritoneum and retroperitoneum have recently been identified;[4,5] these extra-gastrointestinal tumours comprised 6.7% of a series of 1004 GISTs from the Armed Forces Institute of Pathology.[3]

The tumours present clinically as a mass (two-thirds exceed 50 mm at presentation), or with pain or bleeding, or symptoms of metastasis. There is an increased incidence of GISTs including multiple small intestinal tumours in patients with von Recklinghausen's neurofibromatosis (NF-1), possibly associated with interaction between the NF-1 gene product and *c-kit*,[6] and GIST is occasionally familial and associated with a germline *c-kit* or, more rarely, PDGFRA mutation, as discussed below. Some patients have second cancers, and some epithelioid gastric stromal tumours are associated with paraganglioma and pulmonary chondroma in Carney's triad.

NATURE AND DIFFERENTIATION

Interstitial cells of Cajal are involved in regulation of gastrointestinal motility by pacemaker activity and also have a role in muscle relaxation.[7] They are slender cells with ovoid nuclei and scanty cytoplasm, mostly located in the Auerbach's myenteric plexus of the stomach, small intestine and colon. Interstitial cells of Cajal surround autonomic ganglia and extend processes between muscle cells near the plexuses. Possibly in relation to origin from a mesenchymal precursor capable of divergent differentiation,[8] interstitial cells of Cajal have incomplete features of both neural and myoid differentiation as shown by immunohistochemistry and ultrastructure. Embryologically, interstitial cells of Cajal appear not to migrate in with nerves but are thought to develop locally in mesenchyme. Immunohistochemical and molecular genetic studies have shown interstitial cells of Cajal to express CD117 (which is required for development of the interstitial cell system) and usually also CD34 in a small subpopulation,[9] although most CD34 positive cells in this context are fibroblasts.

The distribution of interstitial cells of Cajal varies throughout the gastrointestinal tract and correlates with the observed incidence of GISTs in the different regions. In the gastric fundus, they are scanty and mostly occur in the circular muscle layer. In the gastric body and antrum, they are located in the plexus and circular muscle, and in the antrum there is a further plexus in the submucosa. In the small intestine, interstitial cells of Cajal are found mostly in Auerbach's plexus and also in the circular muscle. In the large intestine, they are most frequent in the transverse colon, especially in the taeniae. Interstitial cells of Cajal can appear enlarged or hypertrophic and even dysplastic adjacent to a GIST.[10] However, the occurrence of similar neoplasms outside the gastrointestinal tract, where interstitial cells of Cajal are not known to occur, remains unexplained.

By morphology, immunohistochemistry and electron microscopy, GISTs vary from undifferentiated or uncommitted to showing partial myoid or neural differentiation and, because of their shared CD117 immunoreactivity, it has become accepted that the differentiation is towards interstitial cells of Cajal. However, as pointed out by Rosai,[11] this is to confuse 'histogenesis' with phenotype, since the CD117 positivity in GISTs is due to gain-of-function mutation, *i.e.* it is expressed by a different mechanism than that in interstitial cells of Cajal.

MORPHOLOGY

GIST display a wide range of morphological forms, with spindle, epithelioid and rarely pleomorphic forms, in a variety of patterns and with modifications due to stromal features (Figs 1–6). They vary in diameter from 10 to > 200 mm, and can be submucosal, intramuscular or subserosal in location. Grossly, they are solid or cystic with variable haemorrhage and necrosis, including mucosal ulceration and cavitation.

The two principal cell forms are spindled and epithelioid, which can co-exist in varying proportions. About 70% of gastric GISTs, and the majority of most of those in the rest of the bowel, are spindle-celled tumours.[12,13] The spindle cells are relatively short, are often uniform, and have tapered nuclei with amphophilic or eosinophilic slightly fibrillary cytoplasm. They form cellular sheets and fascicles with whorled, storiform or palisaded patterns. In epithelioid GISTs, the cells have more abundant cytoplasm, with perinuclear glycogen and well-defined cell borders. Clear cell, signet ring cell, oncocytic and plasmacytoid variants occur. The number of mitoses varies from none to many, but pleomorphic tumours are rare; they can display haemorrhage and necrosis. The stroma is scanty, but fibrous septa sometimes delineate tumour nests in an organoid pattern. Myxoid or cystic change or hyalinisation is sometimes seen, and there can be a variable lymphoplasmacytic inflammatory infiltrate, and sometimes osteoclast-like multinucleated giant cells.

IMMUNOHISTOCHEMISTRY

Early immunohistochemical studies aimed to prove supposed smooth muscle, neural or dual differentiation in GISTs, and to relate immunophenotype to behaviour. Varying proportions were shown to have actin and desmin, with fewer cases displaying S100 protein positivity.[14] Significant numbers remained, however, with no specific markers. GANTs were variably immunoreactive for neuron-specific enolase, neurofilaments, synaptophysin and S100 protein. By 1994, CD34 was shown to be a reliable marker for the majority of GISTs,[15] and from 1998 CD117 positivity became a defining feature.[10,16]

CD117 (kit), the product of the *c-kit* gene, is expressed among normal cells in interstitial cells of Cajal, mast cells, melanocytes, a variety of epithelia (breast, salivary gland, sweat gland, nephron), fetal endothelial cells and a subset of CD34-positive haemopoietic stem cells. Staining is usually cytoplasmic, but can be membranous in mast cells, melanocytes and germ cells (Figs 7 and 8). With immunohistochemistry, CD117 is positive (diffuse

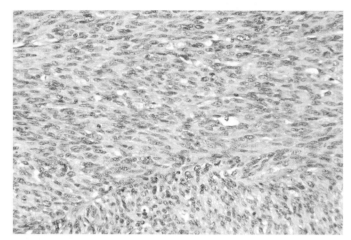

Fig. 1 Spindle cell GIST with fascicles and sheets of relatively uniform cells.

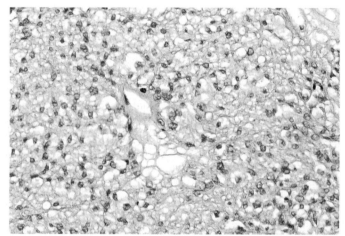

Fig. 3 Epithelioid GIST showing vacuolated cytoplasm.

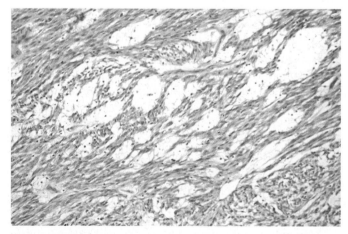

Fig. 5 Myxoid change in the stroma of GIST, the appearances resembling myxoid smooth muscle tumour.

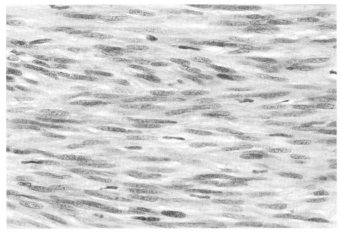

Fig. 2 The cells have elongated, slightly sinuous nuclei with blunt or pointed ends and occasional paranuclear vacuoles. There is a variable amount of cytoplasm giving focally an impression of overlapping nuclei.

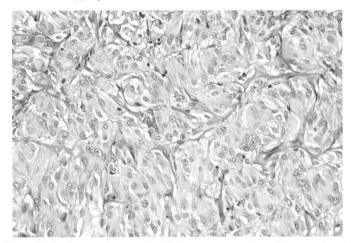

Fig. 4 Epithelioid GIST displaying organoid arrangement with uniform nests of cells.

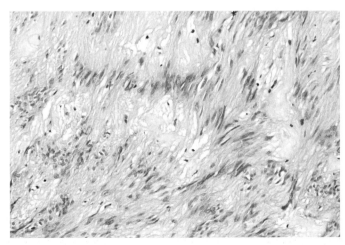

Fig. 6 Foci of palisading are frequently found in GISTs.

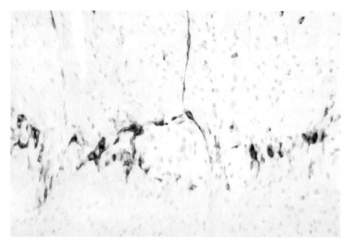

Fig. 7 In muscularis propria of stomach, immunostaining for CD117 reveals interstitial cells of Cajal, surrounding ganglia in Auerbach's plexus and with cytoplasmic processes extending into muscle layer.

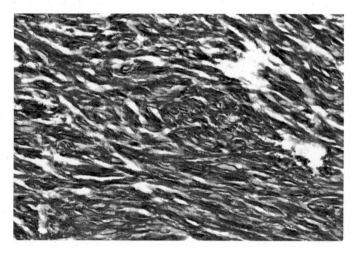

Fig. 8 CD117 positivity in GIST is typically intense and diffuse.

cytoplasmic staining with membranous accentuation) in nearly all GISTs with spindle cell or epithelioid morphology, though less intensely in the latter.[16,17] A small number of otherwise typical GISTs are CD117 negative,[18] and immunoreactivity for CD117 is sometimes lost in metastases. Smooth muscle tumours (smooth muscle actin and desmin positive) and Schwannomas (S100 protein positive) are negative for CD117. Dermatofibrosarcoma protuberans, haemangiopericytoma, sclerosing well-differentiated liposarcoma, angiosarcoma and Kaposi sarcoma are occasionally focally positive. Other CD117-positive non-gastrointestinal tumours include melanoma and clear cell sarcoma (about a third of cases), small cell lung carcinoma, Ewing's sarcoma, anaplastic large cell lymphoma, Reed–Sternberg cells, acute myeloid leukaemia, seminoma, glioma and endometrial carcinoma.[19]

Several commercial antibodies to CD117 are available, with varying specificity and sensitivity.[19] It is necessary, therefore, when evaluating a tumour (or the literature) to be aware of the range of immunostaining expected for each reagent. For example, using the rabbit polyclonal CD117 antibody marketed by Santa Cruz Biotechnology (C-19, sc-168), positivity is essentially confined to GISTs, among the similar tumours in the differential diagnosis. The rabbit polyclonal antibody A4502, manufactured by Dako, is more sensitive but has been reported to stain the cytoplasm of reactive and neoplastic fibroblasts and myofibroblasts, including some examples of fibromatosis, and solitary fibrous tumour, so that its interpretation in the context of GIST diagnosis requires caution. In addition, staining varies with the technical details of the immunohistochemical reaction, including dilutions and use of antigen retrieval. This is particular important because of the introduction of effective anti-c-kit receptor therapeutic agents, use of which depends on demonstration of CD117 immunoreactivity.

CD34 is positive in 47–100% of GISTs,[10,17] and its expression varies with location within the gastrointestinal tract. Miettinen et al.[17] found, among CD117 positive-tumours, 100%, 90%, 47%, 65%, 96%, and 64% of cases to be CD34 positive in oesophagus, stomach, small intestine, colon, rectum and extra-intestinal locations, respectively. Tumours which are CD34 positive are almost always CD117 positive and most CD34 negative tumours are CD117 positive.[20] CD34 is perhaps more often negative in malignant GISTs. CD34 is also positive in occasional smooth muscle tumours including epithelioid variants.

Smooth muscle actin is found only focally in 0–47% of GISTs in an inverse frequency of expression to that of CD34 (the two sometimes showing a mosaic distribution).[17] h-Caldesmon is positive in about 80% of GISTs, and calponin in about 25%.[21] Desmin is focally positive in up to 20% of tumours of oesophagus and omentum/peritoneum, and in a small proportion (< 5%) of benign (but not in malignant) GISTs in stomach and small intestine.

Cytokeratins are usually absent but are occasionally seen in malignant epithelioid GISTs. A few GISTs have presumed neurogenic differentiation, with positivity for S100 protein (especially in small bowel tumours; in 10–15%), PGP9.5 and neuron-specific enolase and some of these additionally express smooth muscle actin, implying both neurogenic and myoid differentiation.

ULTRASTRUCTURE

A minority of GISTs show focally incomplete features of smooth muscle differentiation, with arrays of cytoplasmic intermediate filaments and dense bodies. They differ from true smooth muscle tumours, which have uniform myofilaments, with surface specialisations of pinocytotic vesicles or caveolae, attachment plaques and interrupted external lamina, and which lack neuroendocrine features. Many GISTs show supposed neuronal differentiation with interdigitating neurite-like cytoplasmic processes that contain microtubules, smooth endoplasmic reticulum, and intermediate filaments. Dense core neuroendocrine granules, some of which are also associated with a prominent Golgi apparatus, and synapse-like structures have been described but these are not a usual feature of interstitial cells of Cajal, and might represent entrapped autonomic nerves. There are numerous mitochondria and occasional cell-to-cell junctions (including with smooth muscle cells and neurones). A recent study[22] has suggested that gastric and omental GISTs are ultrastructurally similar and have better developed features of myoid differentiation; those of small intestine and colon resemble each other, although colonic GIST appear more primitive. Finally, some GISTs, including CD117/CD34 positive cases, show no ultrastructural differentiation.

Skeinoid fibres, which are amorphous PAS-positive foci of haphazardly arranged modified collagen fibres with a periodicity of 45 nm, are seen rarely, and usually in (small) intestinal or duodenal tumours.[23]

GENETICS

The *c-kit* proto-oncogene, located on chromosome 4q11-21, encodes a type-III receptor tyrosine kinase (TK) protein (CD117) of the immunoglobulin supergene family. This receptor is a member of the same subfamily as receptors for platelet-derived growth factors (PDGFRA, PDGFRB) and colony-stimulating factor 1 (MCSF1R). The kit protein has a molecular weight of 145 kDa, and consists of 976 amino acids, with an extracellular domain (497 amino acids) with five Ig-like regions, a transmembrane domain (23 amino acids), and an intracellular (cytoplasmic) TK domain, split by a hydrophilic insert, with an ATP binding site.[24] The extracellular receptor ligand for kit is stem cell factor (scf), an early haematopoietic growth factor; the scf–kit system also plays a role in proliferation and differentiation of melanocytes, erythrocytes, germ cells, mast cells and interstitial cells of Cajal.[25] The ligand binding in the external domain activates the internal tyrosine kinase by homodimerisation, resulting in transfer of the terminal phosphate group from ATP to the hydroxyl group on a tyrosine residue in the cell. This leads to phosphorylation of other proteins and activation of signal transduction cascades which regulate cell proliferation, apoptosis, chemotaxis, and adhesion.[26]

In GISTs, somatic gain of function (constitutive phosphorylation) is associated with activating mutations mostly in the juxtamembrane domain at exon 11, found in 21–90% or more of GISTs.[27] This allows activation (phosphorylation) without ligand binding, one possible mechanism for which is ligand-independent dimerisation or oligomerisation. The mutations are found more frequently in malignant GIST, and preferentially in the spindle cell variant[28] and the prognosis is possibly worse in patients with this mutation. Familial and multiple GISTs are associated with a germline mutation at exon 11.[29] Fewer than 10% of GISTs have an alternative somatic mutation at exon 9 (usually in small intestinal GISTs) or exon 13 which encodes the extracellular domain; these cases have lower mitotic counts.[30] Other *kit* mutations occur in the extracellular and transmembrane domains (*e.g.* exon 2, in CML and myelofibrosis) and the exon 17 phosphotransferase domain (in seminoma and mastocytosis). Gene expression profiling studies have revealed that GISTs have heterogeneous gene expression depending on *kit* genotype and anatomical location of the tumour.[31] *kit* mutations have not been found in smooth muscle tumours.

A minority of GISTs lack demonstrable *kit* mutations, but *kit* is nonetheless strongly activated. About 35% (14 of 40) of GISTs lacking *kit* mutations have been shown to have intragenic activation mutations in the related receptor tyrosine kinase, platelet-derived growth factor receptor alpha (PDGFRA).[32] Tumours expressing kit or PDGFRA oncoproteins were indistinguishable with respect to activation of downstream signalling intermediates and cytogenetic changes associated with tumour progression. In a series of 25 CD117-negative but otherwise typical GISTs, five of which arose in omentum or mesentery, 18 tumours had *PDGFRA* mutations (mostly in exon 18), 4 tumours had *kit* mutations and 3 had neither.[33] Thus, *kit* and *PDGFRA* mutations appear to be alternative oncogenic mechanisms in GIST.

A recent gene expression profiling study has shown that the novel gene *DOG1* (which encodes a hypothetical protein) is expressed ubiquitously in gastrointestinal stromal tumours irrespective of *kit* or *PDGFRA* mutation status,[34] which might be useful for diagnosis and for guidance of therapy in kit-negative cases.

There is also in both benign and malignant GISTs deletion or partial loss of the long arms of chromosomes 14 and 22, suggesting a role for additional tumour suppressor genes. Other cytogenetic changes in GISTs include losses in 1p32 and 1p36. Comparative genomic hybridisation studies have shown loss of 14q, 22 (possibly an early event), and 1p and gains of 5q mainly in malignant GISTs.[35,36]

BEHAVIOUR

GENERAL

Malignant GISTs recur locally and spread mainly to adjacent organs, omentum or mesentery, retroperitoneum and liver, and less commonly (0–15%) to lymph node or extra-abdominally to lung and rarely bone. There have been numerous and conflicting attempts to predict behaviour in this heterogeneous group of tumours. However, the distinction between benign and malignant GISTs cannot be made with certainty because: (i) poorly differentiated tumours do not always behave in a malignant fashion; (ii) very small GISTs in some locations have been recorded to metastasise; and (iii) even the blandest looking tumours can recur, especially when large, and sometimes after a very long period (20–30 years) so that life-long follow-up is required.

Proposed prognostic factors have included size, infiltration of mucosa and muscularis propria, mitotic count, ploidy, proliferation markers (PCNA, Ki-67), necrosis, cellularity, pleomorphism and immunophenotype including loss of CD44s.[37] Benign and low-grade tumours are usually diploid, and most high-grade

Table 1 Proposed guidelines for assessing risk in GISTs

	Size (mm)	Mitotic count/50 hpf
Very low risk	< 20	< 5
Low risk	20–50	< 5
Intermediate risk	< 50	6–10
	50–100	< 5
High risk	> 50	> 5
	> 100	Any
	Any	> 10

tumours are aneuploid, but the distinction is insufficiently clear cut for diagnosis. Aneuploidy is, however, related to poor outcome.[38]

No single factor is sufficiently predictive to be used exclusively, but the main prognostic factors identified have been mitotic count and tumour size. Both are continuous variables and authors have taken various cut-off points. Consensus guidelines using combinations of maximum dimension and mitotic count for defining risk have recently been proposed (Table 1).[39] These guidelines do not, however, take account of regional variations and these are considered separately below.

OESOPHAGUS

GISTs account for 25% of oesophageal stromal tumours (and leiomyomas for 70%), and involve the lower third or gastroesophageal junction, predominantly in males. They can be spindled or epithelioid and display the usual variety of patterns. The majority are aggressive; in the series of Miettinen et al.,[40] 9 of 16 patients died of disease including all with tumours larger than 100 mm, and none with tumours < 50 mm. The median survival was 29 months. Smooth muscle tumours are more commonly seen. Leiomyomas occur in a younger age group than GISTs, and mostly in the lower third of the oesophagus. They are intramural, sausage-shaped and lack mitoses; they are indolent even when large (up to 180 mm) but occasionally recur. Oesophageal leiomyosarcomas are large, high-grade malignancies which lack CD117 (but occasionally express CD34) which are uniformly fatal.

STOMACH

Gastric GISTs are more frequent in males, but young patients, especially females, have a better outcome; Persson et al.[41] reported 4 patients less than 26 years old who had metastasising gastric 'epithelioid leiomyosarcomas', involving liver, nodes, peritoneum, and who all survived for 17–48 years. The 5-year survival of patients with gastric GIST is about 40%, with increased survival in completely resected cases. There is no evidence that radical surgery improves survival; the least extensive surgical procedure compatible with complete excision is advisable.

Epithelioid GISTs (formerly leiomyoblastoma or epithelioid smooth muscle tumour) comprise about 11% of gastric GISTs, of which 73–81% behave in a benign fashion.[42] Large tumours in the fundus or cardiac area and posterior wall are more likely to be aggressive.

DUODENUM

Duodenal GISTs are most common in the second part, and 35–50% are malignant.[43] They are cellular, have more than 2 mitoses per 50 hpf and are usually greater than 45 mm in diameter. No tumour < 20 mm or with < 5 mitoses/50 hpf recurred or caused death.[43] Benign-behaving GISTs are more uniform, less cellular, can display an organoid pattern, and have < 2 mitoses per 50 hpf, but the presence of necrosis or epithelioid change lowers the mitotic threshold for malignancy.

JEJUNUM AND ILEUM

There are few studies specifically of small intestinal GISTs, although general series include examples. They have a worse outcome than gastric GISTs, with an overall 5-year survival of about 40% and a 5-year disease-free survival of 20% for the most aggressive tumours. The overall 10-year survival is around 17% in small intestinal tumours.

COLON

GISTs are seen in adults in the sixth decade in the ascending and descending portions of the colon. Except for small subserosal lesions, they are typically transmural tumours with intraluminal and outward-bulging components. Morphologically they are heterogeneous with spindle cells in fascicles, palisades or storiform arrangement, and sometimes an organoid pattern; a minority has a component of epithelioid cells. In the most recent series,[44] tumours smaller than 10 mm did not recur, whereas among larger tumours 20% with minimal mitoses, and all examples with more than 5 mitoses per 50 hpf, metastasised or died of disease.

APPENDIX

GISTs of appendix are rare. Miettinen and Sobin[45] described 4 cases in adult males 56–72 years of age (mean, 63 years). Two tumours occurred in patients who had surgery for appendicitis-like symptoms: one was an incidental finding during surgery for a malignant gastric epithelioid GIST and one was an incidental autopsy finding. A third was polyploid, projecting outward from the proximal part of appendix. Three tumours were partially obliterating nodules, eccentrically expanding the appendiceal wall. All four were spindle cell tumours, and three of them contained skeinoid fibres; none had atypia or mitotic activity (< 1/50 high power fields). Follow-up revealed death from cardiovascular disease in one case (4 years after appendectomy) and liver failure because of malignant gastric epithelioid GIST metastatic to liver in another case 15 years after the appendicectomy.

ANORECTUM

Of rectal GISTs, 32–54% are malignant, the smallest being 16 mm[46,47] but most exceed 50 mm and have > 5 mitoses per 50 hpf. In a series of 144 anorectal GISTs,[48] 54% recurred or metastasised (to liver, lung or bone), sometimes after a long interval. Survival is around 60% at 5 years and 20–50% at 10 years (for patients with curative rather than palliative resections). As in the oesophagus, true smooth muscle neoplasms are more common than GISTs. Leiomyomatous polyps arising from muscularis mucosae are relatively common. True leiomyosarcomas of anorectum are rare, and form polyploid intraluminal masses; only one of eight such patients died of disease in spite of high mitotic counts.[48]

EXTRAGASTROINTESTINAL GISTS

GISTs occur outside the gastrointestinal tract, in locations where interstitial cells of Cajal have not been shown. They possibly arise from a (hypothetical) common precursor cell that gives rise to GISTs or GIST-like neoplasms. Miettinen et al.[4] described 13 omental and 10 mesenteric cases. Omental spindle cell tumours were less cellular and fascicular than leiomyosarcoma and had less cytoplasmic eosinophilia. Mitotic counts were generally low though two had 19 and 26 mitoses per 50 hpf, respectively. The epithelioid tumours were large (100–300 mm). However, none of the patients with omental GISTs died of tumour, with disease-free survival up to 8.5 years. In contrast, 4 of 9 patients with mesenteric spindle or epithelioid cell tumours died including two with a high mitotic count and two with a low count.

Reith et al.[5] described 48 tumours, in 32 females and 16 males, of which 40 involved the omentum or mesentery (these were not analysed separately), and 8 arose in the retroperitoneum, Most were composed of short spindle cells but epithelioid change was present in half the cases. Of the patients, 39% developed metastases or died of disease. In multivariate analysis, more than 5 mitoses per 50 hpf and the presence of necrosis were predictive factors.

It appears that omental GIST can be large but often have low mitotic counts and do well whereas those originating in the mesentery have a worse outcome. In these respects, GISTs of omentum resemble those of stomach, and GISTs of mesentery are more similar to small intestinal tumours.

TREATMENT

Until recently, surgery (adequate but not radical local excision) has been the treatment of choice, with essentially no role for radiotherapy and little for chemotherapy of disseminated tumours. The management of these tumours has been considerably facilitated by the introduction of gene-product targeted therapy, utilising STI571 (imatinib, Glivec), a 2-phenylaminopyrimidine derivative which is a selective inhibitor of c-abl, c-kit, and PDGFR tyrosine kinases. The first case report was published in 2001[49] and large clinical trials are under way in Europe and the US. So far, a number of gastrointestinal stromal tumours that express *c-kit* have shown a response to this new therapy.[50–52] The response is rapid, and relatively free of side effects, but appears to be related to mutational status of the tumour. Thus, the partial response rate is significantly higher in patients with GIST which have juxtamembrane (exon 11) *kit* mutations, than for tumours containing an extracellular (exon 9) *kit* mutation or no detectable mutation of *kit* or *PDGFRA*.[51,53] Treated tumours show necrosis with small pyknotic nuclei and reduced proliferative activity in surviving cells, which are dispersed in a hyalinised or myxoid background. Other drugs with specific effects are currently being evaluated.

DIFFERENTIAL DIAGNOSIS

This includes a wide range of tumours with spindle cell and epithelioid morphology.

SMOOTH MUSCLE TUMOURS

Leiomyomas, which are sometimes multiple, occur in the oesophageal wall and in the submucosa (muscularis mucosae) of colon and rectum, and extramurally in colon (here resembling uterine leiomyoma and ER positive, unlike GISTs). Mural leiomyomas are extremely rare. True leiomyosarcoma scarcely occurs in stomach, but can be found in small intestine, colon and rectum. Although morphologically somewhat resembling GISTs, smooth muscle neoplasms express desmin, smooth muscle actin and h-caldesmon and lack CD117 and (usually) CD34.

INFLAMMATORY MYOFIBROBLASTIC TUMOUR

This affects a younger, often paediatric, age group and is extramural but can extend into the bowel wall. It has fasciitis-like, fascicular and sclerosing patterns with a prominent plasma cell infiltrate. The cells are myofibroblastic, and longer and more tapered than those of GISTs, and variably display smooth muscle actin, desmin and cytokeratin but not CD34 or CD117. A proportion of cases are immunohistochemically positive for ALK 1.

SCHWANNOMAS

Schwannomas occur in the stomach involving submucosa and muscularis propria and rarely in oesophagus or colon. They are sharply demarcated but not encapsulated, and ovoid but can be plexiform. A lymphoid cuff with germinal centres and intralesional lymphocytes can be seen. These benign tumours are diffusely positive for S100 protein and lack muscle markers and CD117.

INFLAMMATORY FIBROUS POLYP

This occurs mostly in small intestine and stomach, usually in adults. It forms a submucosal sessile, later pedunculated lesion with mucosal ulceration, up to 5 cm diameter, composed of stellate and spindle fibroblasts in a hyaline oedematous stroma containing eosinophils and plasma cells. There is perivascular thickening. The fibroblasts are CD34 positive but CD117 negative.

GLOMUS TUMOUR

Glomus tumours occur in the stomach and sometimes oesophagus. They are histologically similar to those in the skin and soft tissue and are CD117 negative.

FIBROMATOSIS

Fibromatosis can involve the mesentery, retroperitoneum or bowel wall. It tends to occur at a younger age, and the tumour is grossly firmer and homogeneous. There are parallel, evenly distributed bland spindle or stellate myofibroblasts with few mitoses, in variably dense collagen, with typical slit-like or small thick-walled muscular vessels and mast cells. CD117 has been reported as positive, depending on the antibody, dilutions and staining conditions, but usually in the cytoplasm only. Smooth muscle actin is positive in about 75% and desmin focally in 50% of cases, but CD34 is always negative and S100 protein usually so. The diagnostic utility of immunopositivity for β-catenin in nuclei of the cells of deep fibromatoses has recently been demonstrated.[54]

SOLITARY FIBROUS TUMOUR

This can occur in the peritoneal cavity and adhere to bowel. It is composed of nondescript spindle cells with a featureless pattern and interspersed collagen fibres often with focal hyalinisation and a mainly peripheral hemangiopericytomatous vascular pattern. Because nearly all cases are diffusely CD34 positive, and because there are protean patterns, solitary fibrous tumour can be confused with GIST. However, the cytomorphology is somewhat different, and solitary fibrous tumours lack CD117 or have only focal weak positivity.

SPINDLE CELL CARCINOMA

Spindle cell carcinoma is usually pleomorphic and can be associated with a more obvious epithelial component. It is often cytokeratin positive (especially with antibodies to high molecular weight cytokeratins), as well as CD34- and CD117-negative.

FOLLICULAR DENDRITIC CELL SARCOMA

Follicular dendritic cell sarcoma has sheets and whorls of cells with ovoid, speckled nuclei and distinct cell membranes, intimately associated with small lymphocytes. The tumour is positive for CD21/35, and often for EMA and S100 protein.

PECOMAS

Tumours of perivascular epithelioid cells (PEComas) occur in the abdomen and can be CD117 and smooth muscle actin-positive. In addition, however, this tumour type expresses markers of melanocytic differentiation.

MESOTHELIOMA

Mesothelioma when sarcomatoid can sometimes enter the differential diagnosis if it involves the bowel, especially in a small biopsy, but this neoplasm has epithelial markers and calretinin and lacks CD34 and CD117.

DEDIFFERENTIATED LIPOSARCOMA

Dedifferentiated liposarcoma is a pleomorphic sarcoma that lacks CD117. It is predominantly retroperitoneal and extramural and an associated or antecedent component of well-differentiated liposarcoma is also seen.

Points for best practice

- GISTs can occur in any part of the gastrointestinal tract but are most common in stomach and small intestine. They can also occur in mesentery, omentum or retroperitoneum without gastrointestinal connection.

- Most are spindle cell tumours but epithelioid cell variants occur especially in the stomach. Other histological features include signet ring, rhabdoid and plasmacytoid cells, palisading, organoid nests, myxoid change, fibrosis with calcification and giant cells, but pleomorphism is exceptional.

- Almost all GISTs show strong diffuse positivity for CD117. About two-thirds are focally positive for CD34, and a smaller number express smooth muscle actin, but desmin and S100 protein positivity are rare. Other markers that can be positive include h-caldesmon and calponin.

- GISTs usually have activating mutations (permitting somatic gain of function) in the *kit* gene, which encodes a type III receptor tyrosine kinase, of which the ligand is stem cell factor and the gene product is CD117 (kit). The most common mutation is at exon 11 in the juxtamembrane domain, but a minority of tumours have mutations at exon 9 or exon 13 in the extracellular domain.

- A small number of GISTs lack *kit* mutations and some of these have intragenic activation mutations in the related receptor tyrosine kinase, platelet-derived growth factor receptor alpha (PDGFRA).

- An estimate of risk (malignant potential) can be made from tumour diameter and mitotic index. Tumours arising in oesophagus, small intestine or colon behave more aggressively than those in the stomach.

- Specific targeted therapy with a selective inhibitor of receptor tyrosine kinases, such as imatinib, can produce a significant therapeutic response in GISTs. Tumours with mutations at exon 11 are more sensitive to imatinib than those with mutations at exon 9.

References

1. Mazur MT, Clark HB. Gastric stromal tumors. Reappraisal of histogenesis. *Am J Surg Pathol* 1983; **7**: 507–519.
2. Lauwers GY, Erlandson RA, Casper ES, Brennan MF, Woodruff JM. Gastrointestinal autonomic nerve tumors. A clinicopathological, immunohistochemical, and ultrastructural study of 12 cases. *Am J Surg Pathol* 1993; **17**: 887–897.
3. Emory TS, Sobin LH, Lukes L, Lee DH, O'Leary TJ. Prognosis of gastrointestinal smooth-muscle (stromal) tumors: dependence on anatomic site. *Am J Surg Pathol* 1999; **23**: 82–87.
4. Miettinen M, Monihan JM, Sarlomo-Rikala M *et al*. Gastrointestinal stromal tumors/smooth muscle tumors (GISTs) primary in the omentum and mesentery:

clinicopathologic and immunohistochemical study of 26 cases. *Am J Surg Pathol* 1999; **23**: 1109–1118.

5. Reith JD, Goldblum JR, Lyles RH, Weiss SW. Extragastrointestinal (soft tissue) stromal tumors: an analysis of 48 cases with emphasis on histologic predictors of outcome. *Modern Pathol* 2000; **13**: 577–585.

6. Kinoshita K, Hirota S, Isozaki K *et al*. Absence of *c-kit* gene mutations in gastrointestinal stromal tumours from neurofibromatosis type 1 patients. *J Pathol* 2004; **202**: 80–85.

7. Huizinga JD, Robinson TL, Thomsen L. The search for the origin of rhythmicity in intestinal contraction; from tissue to single cells. *Neurogastroenterol Motil* 2000; **12**: 3–9.

8. Kluppel M, Huizinga JD, Malysz J, Bernstein A. Developmental origin and Kit-dependent development of the interstitial cells of Cajal in the mammalian small intestine. *Dev Dyn* 1998; **211**: 60–71.

9. Huizinga JD, Thuneberg L, Kluppel M *et al*. W/kit gene required for interstitial cells of Cajal and for intestinal pacemaker activity. *Nature* 1995; **373**: 347–349.

10. Kindblom LG, Remotti HE, Aldenborg F, Meis-Kindblom JM. Gastrointestinal pacemaker cell tumor (GIPACT): gastrointestinal stromal tumors show phenotypic characteristics of the interstitial cells of Cajal. *Am J Pathol* 1998; **152**: 1259–1269.

11. Rosai J. GIST: an update. *Int J Surg Pathol* 2003; **11**: 177–186.

12. Trupiano JK, Stewart RE, Misick C, Appelman HD, Goldblum JR. Gastric stromal tumors: a clinicopathologic study of 77 cases with correlation of features with nonaggressive and aggressive clinical behaviors. *Am J Surg Pathol* 2002; **26**: 705–714.

13. Tworek JA, Appelman HD, Singleton TP, Greenson JK. Stromal tumors of the jejunum and ileum. *Modern Pathol* 1997; **10**: 200–209.

14. Suster S. Gastrointestinal stromal tumors. *Semin Diagn Pathol* 1996; **13**: 297–313.

15. Monihan JM, Carr NJ, Sobin LH. CD34 immunoexpression in stromal tumours of the gastrointestinal tract and in mesenteric fibromatoses. *Histopathology* 1994; **25**: 469–473.

16. Sarlomo-Rikala M, Kovatich AJ, Barusevicius A, Miettinen M. CD117: a sensitive marker for gastrointestinal stromal tumors that is more specific than CD34. *Modern Pathol* 1998; **11**: 728–734.

17. Miettinen M, Sobin LH, Sarlomo-Rikala M. Immunohistochemical spectrum of GISTs at different sites and their differential diagnosis with a reference to CD117 (KIT). *Modern Pathol* 2000; **13**: 1134–1142.

18. Debiec-Rychter M, Wasag B, Stul M *et al*. Gastrointestinal stromal tumours (GISTs) negative for KIT (CD117 antigen) immunoreactivity. *J Pathol* 2004; **202**: 430–438.

19. Gibson PC, Cooper K. CD117 (KIT): a diverse protein with selective applications in surgical pathology. *Adv Anat Pathol* 2002; **9**: 65–69.

20. Seidal T, Edvardsson H. Expression of *c-kit* (CD117) and Ki-67 provides information about the possible cell of origin and clinical course of gastrointestinal stromal tumours. *Histopathology* 1999; **34**: 416–424.

21. Miettinen MM, Sarlomo-Rikala M, Kovatich AJ, Lasota J. Calponin and h-caldesmon in soft tissue tumors: consistent h-caldesmon immunoreactivity in gastrointestinal stromal tumors indicates traits of smooth muscle differentiation. *Modern Pathol* 1999; **12**: 756–762.

22. Yantiss RK, Rosenberg AE, Selig MK, Nielsen GP. Gastrointestinal stromal tumors: an ultrastructural study. *Int J Surg Pathol* 2002; **10**: 101–113.

23. Min KW. Small intestinal stromal tumors with skeinoid fibers. Clinicopathological, immunohistochemical, and ultrastructural investigations. *Am J Surg Pathol* 1992; **16**: 145–155.

24. Blume-Jensen P, Claesson-Welsh L, Siegbahn A *et al*. Activation of the human *c-kit* product by ligand-induced dimerization mediates circular actin reorganization and chemotaxis. *EMBO J* 1991; **10**: 4121–4128.

25. Ashman LK. The biology of stem cell factor and its receptor C-kit. *Int J Biochem Cell Biol* 1999; **31**: 1037–1051.

26. Heinrich MC, Rubin BP, Longley BJ, Fletcher JA. Biology and genetic aspects of gastrointestinal stromal tumors: KIT activation and cytogenetic alterations. *Hum Pathol* 2002; **33**: 484–495.

27. Rubin BP, Singer S, Tsao C *et al*. KIT activation is a ubiquitous feature of gastrointestinal stromal tumors. *Cancer Res* 2001; **61**: 8118–8121.

28. Wardelmann E, Neidt I, Bierhoff E *et al*. *c-kit* mutations in gastrointestinal stromal

tumors occur preferentially in the spindle rather than in the epithelioid cell variant. *Modern Pathol* 2002; **15**: 125–136.

29. Nishida T, Hirota S, Taniguchi M *et al*. Familial gastrointestinal stromal tumours with germline mutation of the KIT gene. *Nat Genet* 1998; **19**: 323–324.

30. Hirota S, Nishida T, Isozaki K *et al*. Gain-of-function mutation at the extracellular domain of KIT in gastrointestinal stromal tumours. *J Pathol* 2001; **193**: 505–510.

31. Antonescu CR, Viale A, Sarran L *et al*. Gene expression in gastrointestinal stromal tumors is distinguished by KIT genotype and anatomic site. *Clin Cancer Res* 2004; **10**: 3282–3290.

32. Heinrich MC, Corless CL, Duensing A *et al*. *PDGFRA* activating mutations in gastrointestinal stromal tumors. *Science* 2003; **299**: 708–710.

33. Medeiros F, Corless CL, Duensing A *et al*. KIT-negative gastrointestinal stromal tumors: proof of concept and therapeutic implications. *Am J Surg Pathol* 2004; **28**: 889–894.

34. West RB, Corless CL, Chen X *et al*. The novel marker, DOG1, is expressed ubiquitously in gastrointestinal stromal tumors irrespective of KIT or PDGFRA mutation status. *Am J Pathol* 2004; **165**: 107–113.

35. Sarlomo-Rikala M, El-Rifai W, Lahtinen T *et al*. Different patterns of DNA copy number changes in gastrointestinal stromal tumors, leiomyomas, and Schwannomas. *Hum Pathol* 1998; **29**: 476–481.

36. Derre J, Lagace R, Terrier P, Sastre X, Aurias A. Consistent DNA losses on the short arm of chromosome 1 in a series of malignant gastrointestinal stromal tumors. *Cancer Genet Cytogenet* 2001; **127**: 30–33.

37. Montgomery E, Abraham SC, Fisher C *et al*. CD44 loss in gastric stromal tumors as a prognostic marker. *Am J Surg Pathol* 2004; **28**: 168–177.

38. Lerma E, Lee SJ, Tugues D *et al*. Ploidy of 36 stromal tumors of the gastrointestinal tract. A comparative study with flow cytometry and image analysis. *Anal Quant Cytol Histol* 1994; **16**: 435–440.

39. Berman J, O'Leary TJ. Gastrointestinal stromal tumor workshop. *Hum Pathol* 2001; **32**: 578–582.

40. Miettinen M, Sarlomo-Rikala M, Sobin LH, Lasota J. Esophageal stromal tumors: a clinicopathologic, immunohistochemical, and molecular genetic study of 17 cases and comparison with esophageal leiomyomas and leiomyosarcomas. *Am J Surg Pathol* 2000; **24**: 211–222.

41. Persson S, Kindblom LG, Angervall L, Tisell LE. Metastasizing gastric epithelioid leiomyosarcomas (leiomyoblastomas) in young individuals with long-term survival. *Cancer* 1992; **70**: 721–732.

42. Lee JS, Nascimento AG, Farnell MB *et al*. Epithelioid gastric stromal tumors (leiomyoblastomas): a study of fifty-five cases. *Surgery* 1995; 118: 653–660; discussion 660–661.

43. Miettinen M, Kopczynski J, Makhlouf HR *et al*. Gastrointestinal stromal tumors, intramural leiomyomas, and leiomyosarcomas in the duodenum: a clinicopathologic, immunohistochemical, and molecular genetic study of 167 cases. *Am J Surg Pathol* 2003; **27**: 625–641.

44. Miettinen M, Sarlomo-Rikala M, Sobin LH, Lasota J. Gastrointestinal stromal tumors and leiomyosarcomas in the colon: a clinicopathologic, immunohistochemical, and molecular genetic study of 44 cases. *Am J Surg Pathol* 2000; **24**: 1339–1352.

45. Miettinen M, Sobin LH. Gastrointestinal stromal tumors in the appendix: a clinicopathologic and immunohistochemical study of four cases. *Am J Surg Pathol* 2001; **25**: 1433–1437.

46. Haque S, Dean PJ. Stromal neoplasms of the rectum and anal canal. *Hum Pathol* 1992; **23**: 762–767.

47. Tworek JA, Goldblum JR, Weiss SW, Greenson JK, Appelman HD. Stromal tumors of the abdominal colon: a clinicopathologic study of 20 cases. *Am J Surg Pathol* 1999; **23**: 937–945.

48. Miettinen M, Furlong M, Sarlomo-Rikala M *et al*. Gastrointestinal stromal tumors, intramural leiomyomas, and leiomyosarcomas in the rectum and anus: a clinicopathologic, immunohistochemical, and molecular genetic study of 144 cases. *Am J Surg Pathol* 2001; **25**: 1121–1133.

49. Joensuu H, Roberts PJ, Sarlomo-Rikala M *et al*. Effect of the tyrosine kinase inhibitor STI571 in a patient with a metastatic gastrointestinal stromal tumor. *N Engl J Med* 2001; **344**: 1052–1056.

50. Demetri GD, von Mehren M, Blanke CD *et al*. Efficacy and safety of imatinib mesylate in advanced gastrointestinal stromal tumors. *N Engl J Med* 2002; **347**: 472–480.

51. Heinrich MC, Corless CL, Demetri GD *et al*. Kinase mutations and imatinib response in patients with metastatic gastrointestinal stromal tumor. *J Clin Oncol* 2003; **21**: 4342–4349.

52. Duensing A, Heinrich MC, Fletcher CD, Fletcher JA. Biology of gastrointestinal stromal tumors: KIT mutations and beyond. *Cancer Invest* 2004; **22**: 106–116.

53. Debiec-Rychter M, Dumez H, Judson I *et al*. Use of c-KIT/PDGFRA mutational analysis to predict the clinical response to imatinib in patients with advanced gastrointestinal stromal tumours entered on phase I and II studies of the EORTC Soft Tissue and Bone Sarcoma Group. *Eur J Cancer* 2004; **40**: 689–695.

54. Montgomery E, Torbenson MS, Kaushal M, Fisher C, Abraham SC. Beta-catenin immunohistochemistry separates mesenteric fibromatosis from gastrointestinal stromal tumor and sclerosing mesenteritis. *Am J Surg Pathol* 2002; **26**: 1296–1301.

Malcolm R. Alison Matthew J. Lovell
Natalie C. Direkze Richard Poulsom

6

Adult stem cells and transdifferentiation

In 1998, two papers were published describing the *in vitro* growth of human embryonic stem (ES) cells derived either from the inner cell mass (ICM) of the early blastocyst or the primitive gonadal regions of early aborted fetuses. Work on murine embryonic stem cells over many years had already established the amazing flexibility of ES cells, essentially able to differentiate into almost all cells that arise from the three germ layers (pluripotentiality). The realisation of such versatility in human cells has, of course, resulted in the field of stem cell research going into overdrive, with the belief that stem cell research will deliver a revolution in terms of how we treat cardiovascular, renal and neurodegenerative disease, cancer, diabetes and the like. However, many people believe that early human embryos should be accorded the same status as a sentient being and thus their 'harvesting' for stem cells is morally unjustifiable. With this in mind, other sources of malleable stem cells have been sought. In the adult, organ formation and regeneration was thought to occur through the action of organ- or tissue-restricted stem cells (*i.e.* haematopoietic stem cells making blood, gut stem cells making gut). However, we now believe that stem cells from one organ system, for example the haematopoietic compartment, can generate the differentiated cells within

Malcolm R. Alison DSc FRCPath (for correspondence)
Professor, Centre for Diabetes and Metabolic Medicine, Institute of Cell and Molecular Science, 4 Newark Street, Whitechapel, London E1 2AT, UK (E-mail: m.alison@qmul.ac.uk) Tel: +44 (0)207 882 2357

Matthew J. Lovell MBBS BSc MRCP
Clinical Research Fellow, Histopathology Unit, Cancer Research UK, 44 Lincoln's Inn Fields, London WC2A 3PX, UK

Natalie C. Direkze MA MBBS MRCP
Clinical Research Fellow, Histopathology Unit, Cancer Research UK, 44 Lincoln's Inn Fields, London WC2A 3PX, UK

Richard Poulsom PhD DSc FRCPath
Professor, Histopathology Unit, Cancer Research UK, 44 Lincoln's Inn Fields, London WC2A 3PX, UK

another organ system, such as the liver, brain or kidney – a process termed 'transdifferentiation' or plasticity. Thus, certain adult stem cells may turn out to be as versatile as ES cells and so also be useful in regenerative medicine. In this chapter, we summarise the important attributes of stem cells from a variety of sources, clarify the terms used and try and get beyond the hype that so often accompanies apparent new 'breakthroughs' in medical research. We also emphasise the relevance of stem cell biology to metaplasia, the process of fibrosis and to the development and treatment of cancer.

STEM CELL RESEARCH COMES OF AGE

Morbidity and mortality as a result of malfunctions in vital organs plague, especially, the most technologically advanced societies. Because of a dearth of transplantable organs there is a growing hope that stem cells may be the answer to mankind's prayer to be able to replace tissues worn out by old age and ravaged by disease. Indeed, it is impossible to open a newspaper today without seeing yet another apparent 'breakthrough' in stem cell research; the more optimistic hoping for an elixir of life – the promise of immortality.

Legislation regarding the use of ES cells varies around the globe. In countries like the UK and Australia, new cell lines can be created from spare embryos with the uncompensated permission of the donors. However, in the US at the moment, in a compromise between proponents and critics of ES cell research, federal funds (taxpayers' money) can only be used on ES cell lines created before 9 August 2001; reasoning that such cells while exhibiting pluripotency have not the ability to develop into a whole human being, thus the sanctity of human life is not compromised by their use. However, many of these 'approved' cell lines are no longer available, and most of the others were grown in the presence of mouse feeder cells (to supply essential growth factors), exposing human cells to potentially pathogenic murine viruses and proteins, thus rendering them unsuitable for clinical therapies. In the UK, the Human Fertilization and Embryology Authority (HFEA: <http://hfea.gov.uk/Home>) licences and monitors all human embryo research, including using embryos for stem cell extraction. Moreover, on 19 May 2004 the world's first stem cell bank opened in the UK, jointly overseen by the MRC and BBSRC (<http://www.ukstemcellbank.org.uk/>), acting as a repository and potential supplier of all types of human stem cells, not just embryonic but also those derived from fetal and adult tissues and discarded cord blood. Though no one really doubts that ES cells are likely to be the most flexible of all stem cells, the ethical issues surrounding their use and concerns over their potentially unrestricted growth have prompted the search for alternative adult sources.

ADULT STEM CELLS

According to some (Michael Fumento; <http://www.fumento.com/biotech/stemcell.html>), there is a 'stem cell cover-up', a deliberate attempt to downplay the therapeutic value of adult stem cells in order to divert more attention (money) to ES research; it has been called 'stem cell wars'. While we do not wish to get into this conspiracy theory, adult stem cells, in particular bone marrow transplants, have been used to treat the likes of leukaemia since the 1980s.

PROPERTIES OF ADULT STEM CELLS

A hierarchy of potential

As we have already seen, the appeal of ES cells is the fact that they are pluripotent, able to differentiate into almost all cells that arise from the three germ layers, but not the embryo because they are unable to give rise to the placenta and supporting tissues. On the other hand, most adult tissues have multipotential stem cells, cells capable of producing a limited range of differentiated cell lineages appropriate to their location, *e.g.* small intestinal stem cells can produce all four indigenous lineages (Paneth, goblet, absorptive columnar and enteroendocrine), central nervous system (CNS) stem cells have trilineage potential generating neurons, oligodendrocytes and astrocytes,[1] while the recently discovered stem cells of the heart can give rise to cardiomyocytes, endothelial cells and smooth muscle.[2] However, describing tissue-based stem cells as 'multipotential' may be incorrect if, as it appears, some adult stem cells when removed from their usual location can transdifferentiate into cells that arise from any of the three germ layers (so-called plasticity). The least versatile are unipotential stem cells, cells capable of generating one specific cell type. Into this category, we could place epidermal stem cells in the basal layer of the interfollicular epidermis that produce only keratinised squames and certain adult hepatocytes that have long-term repopulating ability.[3]

Self-maintenance

Stem cells are usually relatively undifferentiated, not having the functional specialisations of the progeny that they give rise to. Perhaps the single most important property of stem cells is their ability to self-renew. They are normally located in a restrictive environment called a niche (*Fr.* recess, see Fig. 1a), and in a tissue such as the small intestine they are found close to the crypt base at the origin of a bidirectional flux (Fig. 1b). In the heart, they are located in areas of least haemodynamic stress. Though comprising only a small percentage of a tissue's total cellularity, stem cells maintain their numbers if, on average, each stem cell division gives rise to one replacement stem cell and one transit amplifying cell (an asymmetric cell division). The interactions with the stem cell niche are crucial to this process and the controlling factors are rapidly becoming elucidated. In the *Drosophila* ovariole, a stem cell niche known as the 'germarium' has been defined, and here germline stem cell (GSC) number is maintained by the close apposition of GSCs with cap cells; Armadillo (fly β-catenin) and decapentaplegic (DPP; a homologue of mammalian bone morphogenetic proteins [BMPs]) signalling are involved.[4] Likewise, in the *Drosophila* testis, GSC number is strictly controlled by the interaction with so-called hub cells[5] – in both the ovariole and testis, disruption of DPP signalling and/or Armadillo/adenomatous polyposis coli (APC) interactions can result in supernumerary GSCs due to alterations in the orientation of the mitotic axes (see Fig. 1a). In mammals too, cadherin/catenins and BMP signalling are also involved in the maintenance of haematopoietic stem cell number through interactions with osteoblasts.[6]

Proliferation, clonogenicity and genomic integrity

Stem cells are slowly cycling but highly clonogenic. Teleologically, it would seem prudent to restrict stem cell division because DNA synthesis can be error-

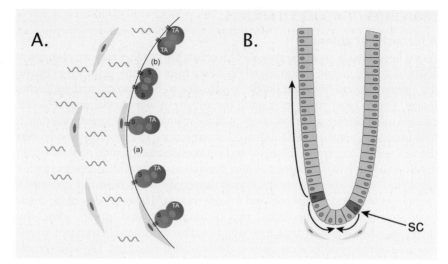

Fig. 1 The stem cell niche. (A) The niche (micro-environment) is likely to control many facets of stem cell behaviour including the rate of division, the orientation of mitotic axes and the type of division (symmetric [both daughters either remain as stem cells {S} or both become transit amplifying {TA} cells] versus asymmetric). The effectors are likely to be secreted soluble factors (growth factors), integral membrane proteins that require cell–cell contact such as the receptor Notch and its ligand Delta, and cell adhesion molecules such as integrins that maintain contact with the extracellular matrix. (B) In the small intestine, the stem cells are at cell positions 3 and 4 (counting from the bottom), and cell flux is largely unidirectional towards the crypt orifice, though some stem cell progeny move downwards to become Paneth cells. The niche is in the underlying lamina propria and the subepithelial myofibroblasts are responsible for Wnt signalling, *etc.*

prone. Thus, in many tissues, stem cells divide less frequently than transit amplifying cells: in the intestine, stem cells cycle less frequently than the more luminally located transit amplifying cells, and in the human epidermis the integrin-bright cells have a lower level of proliferation than the other basal cells. In hair follicles, the hair shaft and its surrounding sheaths are produced by the hair matrix that is itself replenished by the bulge stem cells. As befits true stem cells, the bulge cells divide less frequently but are more clonogenic than the transit amplifying cells of the hair matrix. Combined to an infrequently dividing nature, stem cells would also appeared to have devised a strategy for maintaining genome integrity. Termed the 'immortal strand' hypothesis or Cairns' hypothesis, stem cells can apparently designate one of the two strands of DNA in each chromosome as a template strand, such that in each round of DNA synthesis while both strands of DNA are copied, only the template strand and its copy is allocated to the daughter cell that remains a stem cell.[7] Thus, any errors in replication are readily transferred (within one generation) to transit amplifying cells that are soon lost from the population. Such a mechanism probably accounts for the ability of stem cells to be 'label retaining cells' after injection of DNA labels when stem cells are being formed.

Adult stem cell identity

In many tissues and organs, the identity of the stem cells has remained either elusive or at least equivocal, thus the search for true 'stem cell markers' has become frenetic. Some have argued that stem cell markers are like the spots on a Dalmatian dog, useful for identification, but not appearing to play an essential role in dog (stem cell) function. However, in the bone marrow, the recognition of cells with the properties of self-renewal and multilineage differentiation potential is well advanced. In fact such cells were recognised operationally back in 1961 by Till and McCulloch as cells that gave rise to multilineage haematopoietic colonies in the spleen (colony forming units – spleen [CFU-S]). In the human bone marrow, the sialomucin CD34 is a haematopoietic cell surface antigen that has been exploited extensively for the selection of long-term repopulating cells with multilineage potential, though not all HSCs express this marker. In the mouse, HSCs are recognised also as KLS cells (c-kit$^+$lin$^-$Sca-1$^+$). An alternative method of enriching for HSCs exploits the fact that some cells have evolved a cellular protection mechanism against toxic metabolites and xenobiotics. This mechanism involves the expression of efflux pumps that belong to the ATP-binding cassette (ABC) superfamily of membrane transporters, and such cells are able to efflux a combination of Hoechst 33342 and Rhodamine123, thus appearing at the bottom left corner of a dual parameter FACS analysis – hence called the side population (SP). There are SP cells in many other tissues that might well correspond to their multipotential stem cells.[8]

In the basal layer of the interfollicular epidermis, clusters of likely stem cells are highly expressive of melanoma chondroitin sulphate proteoglycan, along with the β-1 integrin, the receptor for type IV collagen (a component of the underlying basement membrane).[9] In the CNS, neural stem cells and probably their transit amplifying descendants express both the intermediate filament nestin and a RNA-binding protein known as musashi 1. Musashi 1 was first identified in *Drosophila* and thought responsible for the asymmetric divisions of sensory organ precursor cells; it may also be a marker for intestinal crypt stem cells.[10]

Molecular control of stem cell behaviour

It appears likely that the local micro-environment, through a combination of cells and extracellular matrix components (the niche), will govern all aspects of stem cell behaviour. In the intestinal mucosa, the pericryptal myofibroblasts that ensheath the crypts serve as niche forming cells secreting Wnt proteins. One of the most striking observations was made through targeted disruption of the *Tcf-4* gene. Tcf-4 is a partner protein for β-catenin, and the heterodimer transactivates a number of genes involved in cell cycle progression: the absence of Tcf-4 results in the small intestinal crypts failing to maintain a proliferative zone.[11] In turn, Wnt signalling is kept in check by bone morphogenetic proteins (BMPs), also produced by pericryptal mesenchymal cells.[12] Paradoxically, activation of the Wnt pathway through mutation of the *APC* gene is the earliest recognisable abnormality in human colonic carcinogenesis.[13] In the CNS and haematopoietic system, a key regulator of stem cell renewal appears to be Bmi1, a member of the *Polycomb* family of transcriptional repressors. Bmi1 targets genes such as $p16^{Ink4a}$ and $p19^{Arf}$, preventing stem cell senescence by respectively maintaining cyclinD/Cdk4 signalling and Mdm2 destruction of p53.[14] Bmi1 is in fact a downstream target of Sonic hedgehog (SHH) *via* the latter's activation of the Gli family of transcription factors. SHH acts on the receptor complex of patched (PTCH) and Smoothened (SMO), blocking the inhibitory influence of PTCH on SMO, resulting in SMO signalling activating Gli and so transcription of its target genes like Bmi1. In the skin, mutations in *PTCH* characterise human nevoid BCC (basal cell carcinoma) syndrome (also known as Gorlin's syndrome), and clearly SHH signalling in follicular outer root sheath cells leads to BCC, a tumour characterised by a marked lack of features of terminal differentiation.[15] The Notch family of receptors is also critical for stem cell self-renewal, particularly so in haematopoietic stem cells;[16] engagement of ligands of the Delta and Jagged families causes cleavage of the intracellular portion of Notch and its translocation to the nucleus where it acts as a transcription factor. Constitutive Notch signalling is a powerful signal for leukemogenesis (reviewed by Attar and Scadden[17]).

STEM CELL DISEASES – METAPLASIA, FIBROSIS AND CANCER

The resurgence in interest in stem cells has reaped dividends in terms of how we understand other diseases. Metaplastic and heterotopic changes from one recognisable tissue phenotype to another are well recognised in histopathology and are mostly in tissues with a high turnover of cells; such changes may result from genetic or epigenetic alterations that affect expression of transcription factors, presumably in stem cells. For example, overexpression of the transcription factor Cdx2 targeted to gastric epithelium results in islands of intestinal metaplasia.[18] Conversely, the absence of Cdx2 expression in cdx2-null:wild-type chimaeric mice results in patches of Cdx2-null gastric phenotype within wild-type colonic mucosa;[19] importantly, the junctional epithelium had the phenotype of small intestinal mucosa despite being of wild-type heritage and so their local stem cell units had adopted a specific relevant programme of differentiation appropriate to their location.

Myofibroblasts are a distinguishing feature of pathological fibrosis, historically regarded as having originated by activation of local parenchymal fibroblasts, and being the primary collagen-producing cells. However, such fundamental concepts regarding organ scarring will have to be reconsidered in the light of recent findings that bone marrow-derived cells contribute to fibrogenesis in both pulmonary[20] and hepatic scarring.[21] Moreover, bone marrow-derived cells are, at least in part, responsible for the tumour desmoplastic response (Fig. 2).[22] Thus, bone marrow may provide a platform for the delivery of anticancer agents.

Since the classic 'initiation–promotion' experiments involving painting carcinogens on mouse back skin,[23] it has been apparent that many cancers, particularly those of continually renewing tissues (blood, gut, skin), are in fact a disease of stem cells since these are the only cells that persist in the tissues for a sufficient length of time to acquire the requisite number of genetic changes for malignant development.[24] Moreover, tumours are heterogeneous populations in which many cells are terminally differentiated (reproductively sterile) or transit amplifying cells with limited division potential, and so it seems that only tumour stem cells are capable of 'transferring the disease'. For example, in human acute myeloid leukaemia, only the CD34+CD38− cells are capable of propagating the disease in immunodeficient NOD/SCID mice,[25]

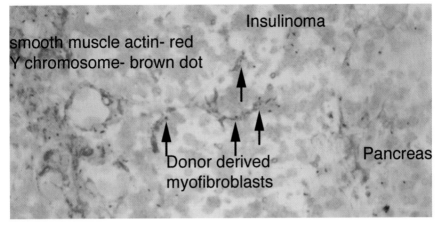

Fig. 2 Mouse model of pancreatic insulinoma demonstrating the contribution of bone marrow to the desmoplastic reaction. This female mouse had a bone marrow transplant from a male donor 2 months beforehand. The tumour (left-hand side) is surrounded by myofibroblasts that express α-smooth muscle actin, and also have a Y chromosome indicating their origin from the bone marrow transplant.

while in human breast cancer, the CD44+ESA+CD24−/low fraction has a similar potential.[26] In the CNS, CD133 appears to be expressed on those cells with the greatest clonogenic potential *in vitro*, again presumably the stem cells.[27] Therefore, there is a growing conviction that successful cancer chemotherapy depends upon eradicating all the stem cells within a cancer.

ADULT STEM CELL PLASTICITY

A large body of evidence now supports the idea that certain adult stem cells, particularly those of bone marrow origin, can engraft alternative locations (*e.g.* non-haematopoietic organs), particularly when the recipient organ is damaged, and transdifferentiate in to cell types with functions appropriate to their new location (Fig. 3). Hence, there is considerable excitement in using haematopoietic stem cells (HSCs) in cell-based therapies and as vectors to deliver therapeutic genes for the correction of diseases such as haemophilia. This is particularly attractive to the clinician because bone marrow stem cells can be readily obtained from patients by simply mobilising HSCs into the peripheral circulation by injection of a cytokine such as G-CSF. Moreover, if a patient's own stem cells were taken for *ex vivo* expansion and directed to differentiate into, say, liver cells or brain cells, no immune rejection problems would arise.

However, before the 'Pro-Life' lobby call for an end to ES cell research, seeing HSCs as the panacea for all ills, it is worth noting that not everyone is convinced of their versatility (reviewed by Alison *et al.*[28]). The reasons for this include the fact that certain instances of so-called plasticity have now been attributed to cell fusion between bone marrow cells (or their macrophage descendants) and cells of the recipient organ; furthermore, several remarkable claims have not been confirmed in other laboratories. Lastly, while a scattering of engrafted cells of haematopoietic origin (but with a phenotype appropriate

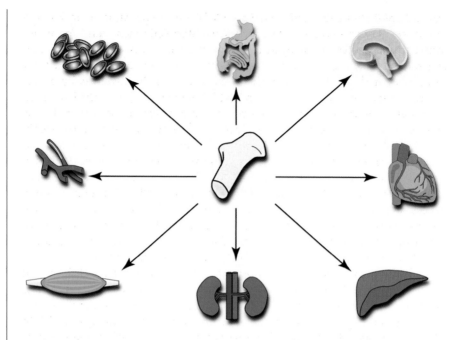

Fig. 3 Adult stem cells, particularly those from the bone marrow, may under certain circumstances migrate to damaged organs, engraft and transdifferentiate into cells of that organ.

to their new location) is often observed in damaged parenchymal organs, these cells appear to have engrafted not as stem cells but either as transit amplifying or terminally differentiated cells, thus their long-term value is questionable. If a bone marrow to, for example, heart axis does exist, one could ask the question: why does bone marrow not seem to act to 'rescue' apparently regeneratively compromised organs such as the damaged heart and brain? There is no easy answer, but the inability to home readily to the damaged tissue may be a crucial factor.

Cell fusion

Claims for adult stem cell plasticity often rely on the appearance of Y-chromosome-positive cells in a female recipient of a bone marrow transplant from a male donor. Alternatively, markers such as LacZ or green fluorescent protein (GFP) have been used, and these techniques are usually combined with lineage markers in attempts to demonstrate there has been a switch in the fate (transdifferentiation) of the transplanted cells. A rapidly growing number of papers suggest that adult bone marrow cells can differentiate into all manner of tissues including skeletal muscle, cardiomyocytes and endothelia, neurones and glia, hepatocytes and bile duct epithelia, renal epithelia and podocytes, and gut mucosal cells and associated myofibroblasts (reviewed by Alison *et al.*[28]). Since most observations have been made in cases of sex-mismatched bone marrow transplantation (donor male bone marrow to female recipient), the obvious step is to examine the cells for the presence of X and Y chromosomes: if fusion was responsible then the donor (apparently) transdifferentiated cell would have an XXXY karyotype rather than XY of a purely transdifferentiated male donor haematopoietic stem cell. The major drawback to this type of analysis is that most are performed on paraffin wax-embedded tissue sections of finite thickness – even in routine 4–6-μm thick sections of male control tissue, the Y chromosome (located usually at the nuclear periphery) is only detected in 50–60% of male cells; thus, the likelihood of 'missing' the extra chromosomes present in a fusion cell is very real. This was not a problem encountered by Tran et al.[29] who analysed almost 10,000 thin buccal cells from 5 female recipients of CD34+ bone marrow cell transplants from male donors. Most significantly, they could detect 98% of Y chromosomes in male control cells and found two X chromosomes in 99% of female control cells. The number of Y- and cytokeratin 13-doubly positive buccal cells in the female recipients ranged from 0.8–12.7%, with only one XXXY cell (0.01%) and one XXY cell (0.01%) detected, both of which could have arisen by fusion. Reasonably, they concluded that bone marrow cells could transdifferentiate directly into buccal cells in the absence of cell fusion.

Diabetes is a major cause of morbidity and mortality, but islet cell transplantation technology is still in its infancy. Thus, the possibility that bone marrow could be used to generate β-cells is very attractive. Adopting a very elegant genetic approach, male mouse bone marrow cells transplanted into lethally irradiated female recipients were found to transdifferentiate, again, without fusion, into pancreatic islet cells possessing many markers of β-cell differentiation and the ability to secrete insulin in response to glucose.[30] However, in undoubtedly the most convincing 'proof of principle' demonstration of the potential therapeutic utility of bone marrow, mice with a metabolic liver disease have been cured.[31] Female mice deficient in the enzyme fumarylacetoacetate hydrolase (fah[-/-], a model of fatal hereditary tyrosinaemia type 1), a key component of the tyrosine catabolic pathway, can be rescued biochemically by 1 x 10^6 unfractionated bone marrow cells that are wild-type for Fah. The salient point to arise from this powerful demonstration of the therapeutic potential of bone marrow cells was that though the initial engraftment was low, approximately one bone marrow cell for every million indigenous hepatocytes, the strong selection pressure exerted by liver failure on the engrafted bone marrow cells resulted in their clonal expansion to eventually occupy almost half the liver. However, it now turns out that the new 'healthy' liver cells in the fah[-/-] mouse contain chromosomes from both the recipient and donor cells, with presumably the donor haematopoietic cell nuclei being reprogrammed when they fused with the unhealthy fah[-/-] hepatocyte nuclei to become functional hepatocytes.[32] The fusogenic partners in the Fah setting have now been identified and are not the HSCs themselves, but are bone marrow-derived macrophages (BMMs) and granulocyte/macrophage progenitors (GMPs).[33,34] In one study, T- and B-cells were found not to be involved, and direct intrasplenic transplantation of either BMMs or GMPs, without lethal irradiation or haematopoietic reconstitution, lead to robust replacement of the Fah null liver with Fah+ hepatocytes.[33] Likewise, Camargo and colleagues[34] came to similar conclusions from a series of experiments including a Cre/lox strategy, involving transplanting bone marrow from mice that expressed Cre recombinase only in the myelomonocytic lineage to Fah null mice that had a floxed β-galactosidase reporter gene; nodules that were positive for both β-galactosidase and Fah indicated that probably Kupffer cells were the fusogenic partners for the Fah-deficient hepatocytes.

Fusion of bone marrow cells has also been found to occur in the normal mouse, not only with hepatocytes, but also with Purkinje cells in the brain and cardiomyocytes.[35] These were very elegant *in vivo* and *in vitro* studies in which a reporter gene was activated only when cells fused. However, unlike the Fah null mouse, no selection pressure (liver damage) was operative, and even after 10 months only 9–59 fused cells/5.5×10^5 hepatocytes were found: importantly, they also found evidence that with time either certain donor genes had been inactivated or eliminated, suggesting genetic instability in such heterokaryons. On the other hand, data from Krause and colleagues[36] suggest that under normal physiological circumstances true transdifferentiation rather than cell fusion prevails. In their study, lethally irradiated female mice that ubiquitously expressed Cre recombinase were the recipients of male bone marrow that would only express EGFP if fusion occurred; at 2–3 months after transplantation, 0.05% of 36,000 hepatocytes were Y-chromosome positive but none expressed EGFP.

On the issue of cell fusion, it would seem reasonable to conclude that, apart from in the liver, heart and Purkinje cells (also skeletal muscle where fusion is the mechanism by which myotubes are generated), there is little evidence for cell fusion between bone marrow-derived cells and parenchymal cells. However, because such a mechanism can occur, makes it mandatory that all investigations at least consider the possibility, notwithstanding the fact that there is nothing inherently wrong in correcting a metabolic deficiency by cell fusion. There is more direct evidence for lineage switching; cultured pancreatic cells can readily differentiate *in vitro* into hepatocytes.[37] Moreover, the induced transdifferentiation commonly occurred directly without cell cycle traverse and involved the vast majority of a pure population of exocrine pancreatic cells – an occurrence that could not involve cell fusion with another cell type. Likewise, when murine HSCs are co-cultured with injured hepatocytes, but separated by a *trans*-well barrier to prohibit cell fusion, differentiation of many of the HSCs to hepatocytes occurred within 2 days.[38]

REPRODUCIBILITY

A major issue that has exercised both protagonists and antagonists of adult stem cell plasticity has focused on the reproducibility of certain remarkable claims. For example, Bjornson *et al.*[39] demonstrated that single LacZ+ neural stem cells could form large colonies (neurospheres) *in vitro* that had all three neural lineages present, and that such neurosphere cells also had haematopoietic potential when transplanted into sub-lethally irradiated mice. An *in vitro* clonogenic assay of the bone marrow from the transplanted mice showed that most (~95%) of the colonies were positive for β-galactosidase suggesting they were of neural stem cell origin. Significantly, cultured neural stem cells neither proliferated nor formed haematopoietic progeny in the same clonogenic assays without prior injection into irradiated host mice, indicating that an appropriate micro-environment was necessary for transdifferentiation. However, another study using a similar protocol to Bjornson and colleagues rigorously tested the haematopoietic potential of murine neurosphere cells and was unable to find any evidence whatsoever of haematopoietic differentiation in a large group (128) of sub-lethally irradiated mice each transplanted with 1 x 10[6] neurosphere cells, which suggested that haematopoietic potential was not a general property of neural stem cells.[40] The therapeutic potential of bone marrow for the treatment of liver disease is also fiercely debated, with some animal models claiming significant and sustained ingress of bone marrow cells that become hepatocytes, while most long-term studies of human liver allografts fail to find any significant chimerism in the graft, despite one report claiming 40% of hepatocytes were derived from the recipient (reviewed by Alison et al.[41]).

Perhaps the most contentious area in this field concerns the myocardium; Orlic et al.,[42] using a murine model of infarction, claim that direct injection of Lin⁻c-kit⁺ HSCs into the peri-infarct zone results in their rapid (within 9 days) transdifferentiation to cardiomyocytes. However, no such conversion was noted by other groups using similar models.[43,44] These latter observations are particularly perplexing given the number of medical centres world-wide, including some in the UK, who are claiming a significant clinical benefit results from the injection of autologous bone marrow to patients with either congestive heart failure[45] or who are recovering from myocardial infarction.[46] Bone marrow is, of course, a well-recognised source of endothelial progenitors, and these may well account for much of the benefits of bone marrow infusion in heart patients, as may also occur in the pancreas. In the pancreas, the role of bone marrow in β-cell renewal is unclear; one study claimed that up to 3% of β-cells could be bone marrow derived shortly after a bone marrow transplant to mice with no obvious pancreatic damage,[30] whereas another study adopting a familiar model of β-cell damage, though noting a beneficial effect of bone marrow transplantation, attributed this to an improved islet blood vasculature.[47]

PATTERNS OF BONE MARROW CELL ENGRAFTMENT

Apart from the murine Fah knock-out liver failure model,[31–34] a notable feature of most plasticity studies is that bone marrow cells do not engraft as stem cells or at least cells with considerable clonal expansion capability. If they did, then one would expect to see patches/columns of bone marrow-derived cells, especially in renewing tissues such as the gut epithelium and epidermis. This has not been the experience in the gut,[48,49] nor generally in epidermis,[50] though a recent study has found evidence for bone marrow cells giving rise to all the cells in a 'epidermal proliferative unit', structures considered to be dependent on the descendants of individual stem cells.[51]

OTHER SOURCES OF ADULT PLURIPOTENT STEM CELLS

In terms of therapeutic potential, there are other sources of adult stem cells that might be amenable to manipulation. These would include cord blood where cells with a wide differentiation repertoire named 'unrestricted somatic stem cells' (USSC) have recently been described,[52] and even the matrix supporting the umbilical cord – so-called Wharton's jelly.[53] There are also the 'multipotent adult progenitor cells' (MAPCs) isolated from mouse, rat and human

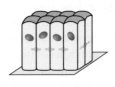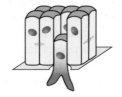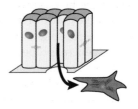

Fig. 4 EMT involves loss of cell–cell adhesion, detachment from underlying connective tissue, induction of motility and acquisition of the mesenchymal phenotype, *e.g.* expression of α-smooth muscle actin and synthesis of collagens.

mesenchymal stem cell (MSC) cultures, that appear capable of differentiating into most, if not all, somatic cell types.[54] Even liposuction waste has 50–100 million stem cells per 250 g, useful for the generation of fat, bone and cartilage. There are also claims that adult cells can be retrodifferentiated and then redifferentiated. Dr Ilham Abuljadayel from TriStem UK Ltd, whose endeavours were widely publicised in *The Sunday Times Colour Magazine* (1 February 2004), claims to be able to turn normal white blood cells into pluripotent stem cells with little more than exposure to a monoclonal antibody against the MHC class II region (CR3/43 from Dako).[55] Furthermore, as reported in the *New Scientist* magazine (9 October 2004), the same antibody has been used to treat successfully 5 patients with aplastic anaemia, seemingly retrodifferentiating *ex vivo* the few marrow cells in these patients back to HSCs that were then re-introduced to the patients. A considerable furore erupted when an online physics journal published with unseemly haste a 'breakthrough' in adult stem cell technology.[56,57] Critics argued that the paper was not rigorously peer reviewed, while the claims made (that pluripotent stem cells can be isolated from adult pancreas) would strengthen opposition to ES cell research. The dermis may also be a source of unusually versatile stem cells; so-called skin-derived precursors (SKPs) have been isolated from the dermal papillae of hair follicles.[58]

EPITHELIAL-MESENCHYMAL TRANSITIONS (EMTS)

EMTs are a very common occurrence during embryonic development, as is the reverse process (MET) – clear examples of cell phenotype plasticity (Fig. 4). Moreover, EMT also occurs in chronic fibrotic disease (*e.g.* in renal interstitial fibrosis), largely mediated by the actions of transforming growth factor-β1 (TGF-β1). It is also likely that EMT occurs in the late stages of tumour progression, allowing epithelial cells to become motile, eventually metastatic cells.[59,60]

SUMMARY

We have reviewed the potential benefits of ES cells and the present legislative framework. We have illustrated that adult stem cells are involved in almost all aspects of tissue homeostasis, they are responsible for normal cell renewal and cited observations that suggest some stem cells, notably HSCs, may have a role in regenerative medicine by virtue of their ability to transdifferentiate. There is also a strong case for channelling more research effort into finding ways to activate the stem cells that do not seem to function appropriately in diseased organs like the brain and heart, and are thus responsible for Western mankind's major causes of morbidity and mortality. Stem cell therapies using either embryonic or adult stem cells may be the solution to the long waiting lists world-wide. On the debit side, cells from the bone marrow may also contribute to organ scarring as seen in liver cirrhosis. Stem cells also exist in tumours, and further characterisation and identification of stem cells in normal tissues might aid in targeting stem cells in cancer.

Points for best practice

- All tissues have stem cells, but in some tissues, notably brain and heart, they do not appear to be activated sufficiently to replace damaged cells adequately.

- In each tissue the control of asymmetric stem cell division, and hence stem cell number, is mediated by signals emanating from the niche, a specialised environment composed of mesenchymal cells and extracellular matrix.

- Multiple signalling pathways compete in the maintenance of stem cell self-renewal and the ultimate differentiation of their progeny.

- Stem cells feature prominently in disease processes; metaplasia illustrates stem cell plasticity, the bone marrow is a source of fibrogenic cells, stem cells are the relevant carcinogen targets and cancers themselves probably all have stem cells.

- Rather than direct transdifferentiation, cell fusion can occur between HSCs and parenchymal cells, reprogramming the HSC genome – nevertheless, a clear sign of the plasticity of the HSC phenotype.

- The derivation of cardiomyocytes from HSCs is controversial in murine models, but the direct intracardiac injection of autologous bone marrow appears to benefit patients with cardiovascular disease.

- Embryonic stem cells are not the only source of versatile stem cells. They can be isolated from bone marrow, peripheral blood, cord blood and Wharton's jelly, liposuction waste, MAPCs from mesenchymal cell cultures, dermal tissue, and may even be derived from retrodifferentiation of peripheral blood mononuclear cells.

References

1. Sanai N, Tramontin AD, Quinones-Hinojosa A *et al*. Unique astrocyte ribbon in adult human brain contains neural stem cells but lacks chain migration. *Nature* 2004; **427**: 740–744.

2. Beltrami AP, Barlucchi L, Torella D *et al.* Adult cardiac stem cells are multipotent and support myocardial regeneration. *Cell* 2003; **114**: 763–776.
3. Alison MR, Poulsom R, Forbes S, Wright NA. An introduction to stem cells. *J Pathol* 2002; **197**: 419–423.
4. Gonzalez-Reyes A. Stem cells, niches and cadherins: a view from *Drosophila. J Cell Sci* 2003; **116**: 949–954.
5. Yamashita YM, Jones DL, Fuller MT. Orientation of asymmetric stem cell division by the APC tumor suppressor and centrosome. *Science* 2003; **301**: 1547–1550.
6. Zhang J, Niu C, Ye L *et al.* Identification of the haematopoietic stem cell niche and control of the niche size. *Nature* 2003; **425**: 836–841.
7. Potten CS, Owen G, Booth D. Intestinal stem cells protect their genome by selective segregation of template DNA strands. *J Cell Sci* 2002; **115**: 2381–2388.
8. Alison MR. Tissue-based stem cells: ABC transporter proteins take centre stage. *J Pathol* 2003; **200**: 547–550.
9. Legg J, Jensen UB, Broad S, Leigh I, Watt FM. Role of melanoma chondroitin sulphate proteoglycan in patterning stem cells in human interfollicular epidermis. *Development* 2003; **130**: 6049–6063.
10. Nishimura S, Wakabayashi N, Toyoda K, Kashima K, Mitsufuji S. Expression of musashi-1 in human colon crypt cells. *Dig Dis Sci* 2003; **48**: 1523–1529.
11. Korinek V, Barker, N, Moerer P *et al.* Depletion of epithelial stem-cell compartments in the small intestine of mice lacking Tcf-4. *Nat Genet* 1998; **19**: 379–383.
12. He XC, Zhang J, Tong WG *et al.* BMP signaling inhibits intestinal stem cell self-renewal through suppression of Wnt-beta-catenin signaling. *Nat Genet* 2004; **36**: 1117–1121.
13. Bienz M, Clevers H. Linking colorectal cancer to Wnt signaling. *Cell* 2000; **103**: 311–320.
14. Park IK, Morrison SJ, Clarke MF. Bmi1, stem cells, and senescence regulation. *J Clin Invest* 2004; **113**: 175–179.
15. Owens DM, Watt FM. Contribution of stem cells and differentiated cells to epidermal tumours. *Nat Rev Cancer* 2003; **3**: 444–451.
16. Karanu FN, Murdoch B, Gallacher L *et al.* The notch ligand jagged-1 represents a novel growth factor of human hematopoietic stem cells. *J Exp Med* 2000; **192**: 1365–1372.
17. Attar EC, Scadden DT. Regulation of hematopoietic stem cell growth. *Leukemia* 2004; **18**: 1760–1768.
18. Silberg DG, Sullivan J, Kang E *et al.* Cdx2 ectopic expression induces gastric intestinal metaplasia in transgenic mice. *Gastroenterology* 2002; **122**: 689–696.
19. Beck, F, Chawengsaksophak K, Luckett J *et al.* A study of regional gut endoderm potency by analysis of Cdx2 null mutant chimaeric mice. *Dev Biol* 2003; **255**: 399–406.
20. Hashimoto N, Jin H, Liu T, Chensue SW, Phan SH. Bone marrow-derived progenitor cells in pulmonary fibrosis. *J Clin Invest* 2004; **113**: 243–252.
21. Forbes SJ, Russo FP, Rey V *et al.* A significant proportion of myofibroblasts are of bone marrow origin in human liver fibrosis. *Gastroenterology* 2004; **126**: 955–963.
22. Direkze NC, Hodivala-Dilke K, Jeffery R *et al.* Bone marrow contribution to tumor-associated myofibroblasts and fibroblasts. *Cancer Res* 2004; **64**: 8942–8945.
23. Stenback F, Peto R, Shubik P. Initiation and promotion at different ages and doses in 2200 mice. I. Methods, and the apparent persistence of initiated cells. *Br J Cancer* 1981; **44**: 1–14.
24. Reya T, Morrison SJ, Clarke MF, Weissman IL. Stem cells, cancer, and cancer stem cells. *Nature* 2001; **414**: 105–111.
25. Bonnet D, Dick JE. Human acute myeloid leukemia is organized as a hierarchy that originates from a primitive hematopoietic cell. *Nat Med* 1997; **3**: 730–737.
26. Al-Hajj M, Wicha MS, Benito-Hernandez A, Morrison SJ, Clarke MF. Prospective identification of tumorigenic breast cancer cells. *Proc Natl Acad Sci USA* 2003; **100**: 3983–3988.
27. Singh SK, Clarke ID, Terasaki M *et al.* Identification of a cancer stem cell in human brain tumors. *Cancer Res* 2003; **63**: 5821–5828.
28. Alison MR, Poulsom R, Otto WR *et al.* Recipes for adult stem cell plasticity: fusion cuisine or readymade? *J Clin Pathol* 2004; **57**: 113–120.
29. Tran SD, Pillemer SR, Dutra A *et al.* Differentiation of human bone marrow-derived cells into buccal epithelial cells in vivo: a molecular analytical study. *Lancet* 2003; **361**: 1084–1088.

30. Ianus A, Holz GG, Theise ND *et al. In vivo* derivation of glucose-competent pancreatic endocrine cells from bone marrow without evidence of cell fusion. *J Clin Invest* 2003; **111**: 843–850.
31. Lagasse E, Connors H, Al-Dhalimy M *et al.* Purified hematopoietic stem cells can differentiate into hepatocytes *in vivo. Nat Med* 2000; **6**: 1229–1234.
32. Wang X, Willenbring H, Akkari Y *et al.* Cell fusion is the principal source of bone-marrow-derived hepatocytes. *Nature* 2003; **422**: 897–901.
33. Willenbring H, Bailey AS, Foster M *et al.* Myelomonocytic cells are sufficient for therapeutic cell fusion in liver. *Nat Med* 2004; **10**: 744–748.
34. Camargo FD, Finegold M, Goodell MA. Hematopoietic myelomonocytic cells are the major source of hepatocyte fusion partners. *J Clin Invest* 2004; **113**: 1266–1270.
35. Alvarez-Dolado M, Pardal R, Garcia-Verdugo JM *et al.* Fusion of bone-marrow-derived cells with Purkinje neurons, cardiomyocytes and hepatocytes. *Nature* 2003; **425**: 968–973.
36. Harris RG, Herzog EL, Bruscia EM, Grove JE, Van Arnam JS, Krause DS. Lack of a fusion requirement for development of bone marrow-derived epithelia. *Science* 2004; **305**: 90–93.
37. Shen CN, Slack JM, Tosh D. Molecular basis of transdifferentiation of pancreas to liver. *Nat Cell Biol* 2000; **2**: 879–887.
38. Jang YY, Collector MI, Baylin SB, Diehl AM, Sharkis SJ. Hematopoietic stem cells convert into liver cells within days without fusion. *Nat Cell Biol* 2004; **6**: 532–539.
39. Bjornson C, Rietze R, Reynolds B *et al.* Turning brain into blood: a hematopoietic fate adopted by neural stem cells *in vivo. Science* 1999; **283**: 534–537.
40. Morshead CM, Benveniste P, Iscove NN *et al.* Hematopoietic competence is a rare property of neural stem cells that may depend on genetic and epigenetic alterations. *Nat Med* 2002; **8**: 268–273.
41. Alison MR, Vig P, Russo F *et al.* Hepatic stem cells: from inside and outside the liver? *Cell Prolif* 2004; **37**: 1–21.
42. Orlic D, Kajstura J, Chimenti S *et al.* Bone marrow cells regenerate infarcted myocardium. *Nature* 2001; **410**: 701–704.
43. Murry CE, Soonpaa MH, Reinecke H *et al.* Haematopoietic stem cells do not transdifferentiate into cardiac myocytes in myocardial infarcts. *Nature* 2004; **428**: 664–668.
44. Balsam LB, Wagers AJ, Christensen JL, Kofidis T, Weissman IL, Robbins RC. Haematopoietic stem cells adopt mature haematopoietic fates in ischaemic myocardium. *Nature* 2004; **428**: 668–673.
45. Perin EC, Dohmann HF, Borojevic R *et al.* Transendocardial, autologous bone marrow cell transplantation for severe, chronic ischemic heart failure. *Circulation* 2003; **107**: 2294–2302.
46. Wollert KC, Meyer GP, Lotz J *et al.* Intracoronary autologous bone-marrow cell transfer after myocardial infarction: the BOOST randomised controlled clinical trial. *Lancet* 2004; **364**: 141–148.
47. Hess D, Li L, Martin M *et al.* Bone marrow-derived stem cells initiate pancreatic regeneration. *Nat Biotechnol* 2003; **21**: 763–770.
48. Korbling M, Katz RL, Khanna A *et al.* Hepatocytes and epithelial cells of donor origin in recipients of peripheral-blood stem cells. *N Engl J Med* 2002; **346**: 738–746.
49. Okamoto R, Yajima T, Yamazaki M *et al.* Damaged epithelia regenerated by bone marrow-derived cells in the human gastrointestinal tract. *Nat Med* 2002; **8**: 1011–1017.
50. Borue X, Lee S, Grove J *et al.* Bone marrow-derived cells contribute to epithelial engraftment during wound healing. *Am J Pathol* 2004; **165**: 1767–1772.
51. Brittan M, Braun KM, Reynolds LE *et al.* Bone marrow cells engraft within the epidermis and proliferate *in vivo* with no evidence of cell fusion. *J Pathol* 2005; **205**: 1–13.
52. Kogler G, Sensken S, Airey JA *et al.* A new human somatic stem cell from placental cord blood with intrinsic pluripotent differentiation potential. *J Exp Med* 2004; **200**: 123–135.
53. Mitchell KE, Weiss ML, Mitchell BM *et al.* Matrix cells from Wharton's jelly form neurons and glia. *Stem Cells* 2003; **21**: 50–60.
54. Jiang Y, Jahagirdar BN, Reinhardt RL *et al.* Pluripotency of mesenchymal stem cells derived from adult marrow. *Nature* 2002; **418**: 41–49.
55. Abuljadayel IS. Induction of stem cell-like plasticity in mononuclear cells derived from unmobilised adult human peripheral blood. *Curr Med Res Opin* 2003; **19**: 355–375.

56. Kruse D, Birth M, Rothwedel J, Assmuth K, Goepel A, Wedel T. Pluripotency of adult stem cells derived from human and rat pancreas. *Applied Physics A*, Published online 26 May 2004.

57. Schiermeier Q, Leeb M. Critics blast 'premature' paper on adult stem cells. *Nature* 2004; **429**: 590.

58. Fernandes KJ, McKenzie IA, Mill P *et al*. A dermal niche for multipotent adult skin-derived precursor cells. *Nat Cell Biol* 2004; **6**: 1082–1093.

59. Prindull G, Zipori D. Environmental guidance of normal and tumour cell plasticity: epithelial mesenchymal transitions as a paradigm. *Blood* 2004; **103**: 2892–2899.

60. Zipori D. The nature of stem cells: state rather than entity. *Nat Rev Genet* 2004; **5**: 873–878.

Andrew R. Dodson
Christopher S. Foster

7

The role of immunohistochemistry in the problematic prostate biopsy

INTRODUCTION

Accurate morphological assessment of prostatic biopsies based upon knowledge of tissue micro-anatomy remains the enduring 'gold standard' of histopathological diagnosis.[1] To this informed understanding may be contributed the 'added value' of immunohistochemistry.[2,3] Although powerful, this technique remains adjunctive and should not be considered as replacing the informed analysis of good histomorphology (Fig. 1). During the past 25 years, since the advent of monoclonal antibody technology,[4] immunohistochemistry has become established as a fundamental technique to assist assessment of pathological tissues. A variety of antibodies (monoclonal and/or polyclonal) and lectins, are routinely employed as probes 'for', 'of' and 'in' prostate cancer. Distinction between the various applications, and hence this terminology, is not semantic since no single reagent is of equal application to answer questions in these distinct areas (Table 1).[5] It is also a generalisation that few, if any, markers are truly pathognomonic for a specific type of cell or tissue. Conventional morphological interpretation of good-quality, thin, tissue sections correctly stained with haematoxylin and eosin and interpreted by

Abbreviations: AAH, atypical adenomatous hyperplasia; AMACR, α-methylacyl-CoA-racemase; AR, androgen-receptor; ASAP, atypical small acinar proliferations (insufficient to confirm diagnosis of malignancy); BCH, basal cell hyperplasia; BrdU, bromodeoxyuridine; EGF, epidermal growth factor; EGFR, epidermal growth factor receptor; HMAR, heat-mediated antigen retrieval; HMWCK, high molecular weight cytokeratin; HGPIN, high-grade prostatic intra-epithelial neoplasia; MVD, micro-vessel density; PAP, prostatic acid phosphatase; PKC, protein kinase C; PCNA, proliferating cell nuclear antigen; PNA, peanut agglutinin; PSA, prostate specific antigen; PTS1, peroxisomal targeting signal; TA, transactivating; TGF-α, transforming growth factor alpha; 5-AR, 5-α-reductase

Andrew R. Dodson MPhil CSci FIBMS
Department of Cellular Pathology and Molecular Genetics, University of Liverpool, Liverpool, UK

Christopher S. Foster MD PhD DSc FASCP FRCPath (for correspondence)
Professor of Cellular Pathology and Molecular Genetics, University of Liverpool, Sixth Floor, Duncan Building, Daulby Street, Liverpool L69 3GA, UK (E-mail: csfoster@liverpool.ac.uk)

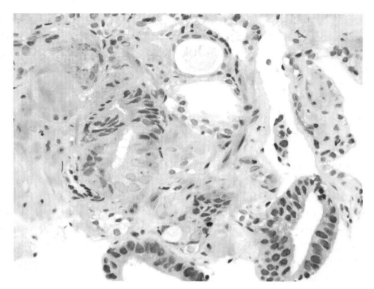

Fig. 1 'The problem': edge of a prostatic needle biopsy and surrounded by unremarkable glands, appearances suggesting *in situ* neoplasia with a few adjacent cells that appear to be invasive carcinoma. The role of immunohistochemical markers is to assist in confirming, or refuting, the diagnosis of malignancy in such situations where morphology, alone, is insufficient.

well-experienced analysts interested in interpreting correctly the morphological appearances remains of paramount importance. The majority of diagnostic problems are associated with confirming (or excluding) prostatic malignancy of epithelial origin; this overview will emphasise that aspect of diagnostic practice. Other applications of immunohistochemistry will be briefly mentioned for completeness and to indicate future likely diagnostic directions.

ANTIBODIES

Immunohistochemistry involves application of antibodies (either monoclonal or polyclonal) to the colourimetric analysis of tissues. Technically, the value of an antibody depends upon its specificity with respect to its cellular target. Whereas polyclonal antibodies recognise multiple sites along a single molecule ('antigen'), monoclonal antibodies recognise a single 'epitope' within a complex antigen.[6] Commonly, but not exclusively, an epitope comprises a short amino acid structure, but may be a defined sequence or array of oligosaccharides or lipids. These may not be simple linear sequences but a spatial distribution resulting from the tertiary structure of the target molecule.

Table 1 Potential antibody applications in prostate cancer

•   Confirmation or exclusion of prostate cancer
•   Identification of prostate cancer within benign prostatic appearances
•   Identification of genotypic sub-types of prostate cancer
•   Prediction of the likely behaviour of a prostate cancer

Both types of epitope (structural and spatial) are critically dependent upon conditions of fixation, whether cross-linking (typically carbonyl-based) or precipitating (typically alcohol-based) and upon the prevailing ionic environment to permit display of the appropriate antigenic or epitopic conformation.

FIXATION

The type and duration of fixation have a profound effect on the results of immunocytochemical staining.[7,8] Satisfactory results can be achieved with formaldehyde-based fixatives and several less common types (*e.g.* Carnoy's or Methacarn). Optimum fixation is essential, and it is standard practice to have protocols to ensure that all specimens are adequately fixed and processed. In routine practice, over-fixation is rarely encountered because turn-around time pressures ensure that specimens are dealt with expeditiously. Under-fixation can, occasionally, cause problems.

ANTIGEN RETRIEVAL

Fixation may cause masking of antigens so that they are no longer recognised by their complementary antibodies. The exact mechanisms that lead to masking are unclear.[9,10] Successful immunostaining often requires reversal of antigen masking, and two methods have been devised to achieve this – proteolytic enzyme digestion and heat mediated antigen retrieval (HMAR). Careful consideration needs to be given to antigen retrieval since it can have profound effects on outcome.

First used in the 1970s, controlled proteolytic digestion of tissue sections enabled the demonstration of a number of otherwise non-reactive antigens.[11] The technique is still employed, although HMAR methods have supplanted digestion for many, but not all, antigens. The key to success lies in choice of a suitable enzyme from a reliable source, and careful control of digestion conditions (which need to be adjusted to account for local differences in fixation and processing).

HMAR has had a major impact on immunohistochemical practice[12,13] since it allows reliable visualisation of a wide range of antigens previously not demonstrable in formalin-fixed, paraffin-wax embedded material. Heat and antigen retrieval solution are the two factors that combine to produce the desired effect, and many comparative reviews have appeared in the literature that can aid in choice.[14–16] Good results can be achieved regardless of heat delivery method provided that a sufficient heating time is employed.[17] Citrate and EDTA are two alternately employed antigen retrieval solutions with which very good results can be produced in the majority of cases.

CONTROLS

As with any immunohistochemical procedure, appropriate controls are of paramount importance and should be the first slides examined before a diagnostician begins to attempt to interpret the staining appearances of a diagnostic problem. Positive control sections allow assessment of whether an antibody is behaving in a predictable manner on a known and frequently-used tissue section, and might alert the pathologist to a possible change in behaviour of a stored antibody or to the altered composition of a new batch of buffer. For such comparisons, it is useful to retain at hand, previous control tissue sections that are dated and stored optimally. Negative controls should also be performed and reviewed assiduously. In these, a section from the test case is stained using the same conditions as those for the positive test sections, with the exception that the primary antibody is replaced by buffer or, preferably, with antibody diluent solution. Such sections will prevent misinterpretation of non-specific staining caused by cross-reaction of the secondary detection system, endogenous pigments, or endogenous biotin where avidin–biotin-based detection has been used.

SPLICE VARIANT PROTEINS

Occurrence of alternative protein structures from an individual gene ('splice variation') is a recent concept appreciated only since the Human Genome Database has become readily accessible. Hitherto, the dictat of 'one gene one protein' was considered to apply to all genes. However, it is now recognised that the majority of genes encode more than one protein by differentially splicing and transcribing various combinations of exons (Fig. 2). It is now understood that different splice variants of some proteins occur at different stages of tissue morphogenesis and during the pathological processes of tissue repair, regeneration or neoplasia. In the interpretation of tissue immunohistochemistry, this concept has two important implications:

1. A monoclonal antibody to a putative protein antigen may not identify the splice variant of that protein if the relevant exon has been spliced-out during evolution of the particular pathological appearances.

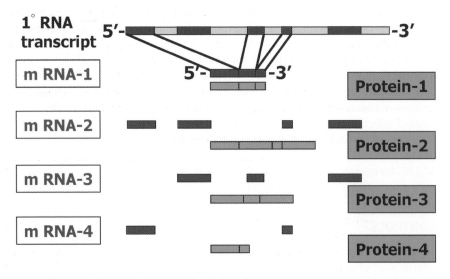

Fig. 2 Schematic diagram of a single gene yielding alternative splice variant proteins leading to differential phenotypic expression, *i.e.* one gene, several different proteins.

2. Unusual staining patterns of an antibody may be due to detection of alternative splice-forms with different intracellular localisation (*e.g.* cytoplasmic versus nuclear) as exemplified by oestrogen receptor proteins lacking the nuclear localisation sequence).

Formerly, it was believed that anomalous patterns of cellular distribution indicated non-functional proteins. However, this view is likely to be too simplistic since it is recognised that some alternatively spliced protein isoforms exhibit different biological properties when distributed to different cellular compartments, thus contributing to altered phenoptyes of affected cells.

CONFIRMATION OR EXCLUSION OF PROSTATE CANCER

The fact that a prostatic specimen contains a malignancy does not always mean *ipso facto* that the malignancy is of prostatic origin. The pathologist should be alert to the possibility that a malignancy within the prostate might be secondary to a primary neoplasm elsewhere (Table 2), and that it is most commonly epithelial in origin (*i.e.* a metastatic carcinoma), although neoplasms arising in mesenchyme (*e.g.* lymphoma) do occur occasionally.

Prostate acid phosphatase (PAP) and prostate specific antigen (PSA) staining of prostate carcinoma tissue are often less intense than that in normal or hyperplastic prostate tissue.[18] In contrast to benign tissue, the majority of reports of prostate carcinoma have demonstrated cell-to-cell and/or field-to-field staining variability for both PSA and PAP. There may also be interstain variability between PSA and PAP from cell-to-cell and/or area-to-area within the same tumour. Decreased PSA and PAP expression in carcinoma have been demonstrated in immunoassays and molecular studies which indicate that the elevated serum levels of PSA and PAP seen in prostate carcinoma reflect an increased volume of carcinoma and/or increased entry into the circulation rather than increased production of PSA and PAP by carcinoma cells.

There appears to be a correlation of staining variability with increasing tumour grade. Image analysis demonstrated no correlation between quantitative PAP extent, or intensity, and grade and suggested that tumour cells' ability to produce PAP is not related exclusively to their ability to form glands.[19] Results of additional studies employing immunoassays and molecular techniques have not been conclusive, although some suggest an inverse relation between tumour grade and tissue PAP and PSA levels.

Table 2 Primary neoplasms that may affect the prostate

- Prostate
- Bladder
- Seminal vesicle
- Ejaculatory duct
- Lymphoma/leukaemia
- Malignant melanoma
- Colon/rectum
- Lung

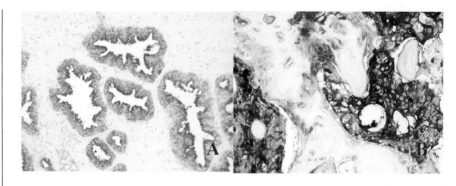

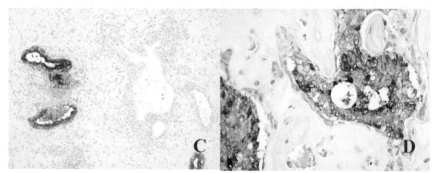

Fig. 3 Expression of PSA in: (A) normal non-malignant prostatic glands; (B) metastatic prostatic carcinoma in bone marrow; (C) absence of PSA expression in a moderately-differentiated transitional cell carcinoma invading prostate; and (D) Comparative expression of PAP in the same bone marrow metastasis as shown in (B).

PROSTATE SPECIFIC ANTIGEN (PSA)

PSA is a 34-kDa, single chain glycoprotein that is 237 amino acids long produced, almost exclusively, by prostatic epithelial cells under regulation by androgens.[20] PSA immunoreactivity (Fig. 3) is most intensely expressed in benign epithelium with staining to a lesser extent in prostatic intra-epithelial neoplasia (PIN) and carcinoma.[21] The number of immunoreactive cells for PSA is not predictive of cancer recurrence. False-positive staining for PSA is less of a problem than is false-negative staining. A few studies[18] of either PAP or PSA staining alone have shown occasional false-negative staining of prostate carcinoma tissue. A large percentage of these cases were high-grade carcinomas or tumours from which only a small amount of tissue was available for study. One *in situ* hybridisation study of PSA mRNA has shown that, even in cases with negative histochemical stains, PSA mRNA may be detected. Occasional staining of urachal remnants, cystitis cystica, cystitis glandularis, and periurethral glands (including Cowper's glands) has also been reported with PSA. Extraprostatic neuroendocrine tumours have consistently been negative. Rare, PSA-positive tumour cells have been reported in bladder adenocarcinoma. Salivary gland tumours have also been shown to stain with PSA. No immunostain is consistently 'best'. While the great majority of prostate carcinomas stain with both PAP and PSA, a few stain with only one or the other, and occasionally with neither. Consequently, it is recommended that both PAP and PSA stains be performed or, if only one is performed and the result is negative, that the other be performed. It is also recommended that, in the case of negative staining of a tumour suspected to be prostate carcinoma, the stain be repeated with increased antibody concentration or incubation time or, if applicable, polyclonal antibodies. Prostate carcinomas with areas of either spontaneous or therapy-induced squamous change can have PAP or PSA positivity in some of the cells with squamous features.[22]

PROSTATE ACID PHOSPHATASE (PAP)

Human PAP is a prostate epithelium-related differentiation antigen. Being the first product of prostatic epithelium to be identified biochemically, and used as a cancer-specific marker, it was a natural target for the generation of polyclonal antibodies to be used in radioimmunoassay and immunohistochemistry to identify prostate cancer cells. However, PAP is not totally prostatic epithelium-specific since it is secreted by a number of other tissues, including those of the reticulo-endothelial system.[23] Although PAP may be secreted by cells of non-prostatic urological origin, it is frequently at a lower level than by prostatic epithelium.[24] Expression of PAP and PSA by prostatic carcinoma cells are not interdependent such that the most important application of PAP immunohistochemistry is to confirm the diagnosis of prostate cancer suggested by morphological appearances (Fig. 3D), but in which PSA staining may be negative or controversial. Staining of urachal remnants, cystitis cystica, cystitis glandularis, or periurethral glands (including Cowper's glands) has been reported and could be misinterpreted as prostate carcinoma. With the exception of staining of neuroendocrine tumours, particularly carcinoid tumours of hindgut origin, bladder adenocarcinoma, and salivary gland tumours, false-positive PAP staining of tumours has not been a significant problem.

5–α-REDUCTASE (5-AR)

Various androgen-metabolising enzymes are present within the prostate,[25] including 5-α-reductase (5-AR). The secretory luminal epithelium of normal and hyperplastic prostatic glands exhibits strong nuclear 5-AR Type 1 reactivity, whereas the androgen-independent basal cell layer variably expresses Types 1 and 2 isoenzymes in nuclear and cytoplasmic compartments. Increased 5-AR reactivity is detected in prostate cancers, particularly those that are high-grade and/or androgen-insensitive.[26–28] Although expression of 5-AR was anticipated to provide a high level of prostatic epithelial selectivity, this expectation has not been realised.

DISTINCTION OF PROSTATE CANCER FROM BENIGN PROSTATIC MIMICS

Once the presence of an epithelial neoplasm within a prostatic biopsy has been established, immunohistochemical assessment can provide valuable adjunct to identify the lesion as a prostate cancer, particularly when morphological criteria that distinguish benign mimics from malignant prostatic epithelial appearances are ambiguous.[1,29] Within this group, markers fall into the two categories of those commonly employed as diagnostic adjuncts, principally to high molecular weight cytokeratins (34βE12) and to α-methylacyl CoA racemase (AMACR or p504s), and those which identify a change in cellular phenotype. The latter are presently less commonly employed in routine diagnostic practice, but may provide additional information with respect to likely tumour behaviour. As in other situations, gain of a marker in malignancy is always more reliable than in one that is diminished or lost during the neoplastic process.

HIGH MOLECULAR WEIGHT CYTOKERATIN (HMWCK)

These are probably the most frequently employed of all antibodies in prostatic diagnostic practice. Originally reported in 1983 to identify prostatic basal

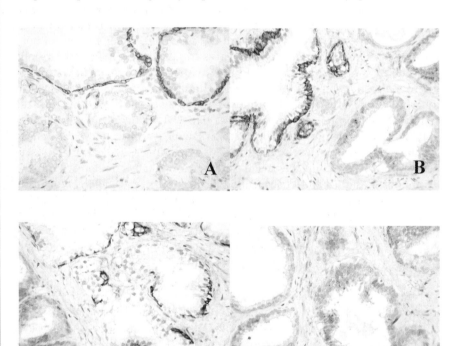

Fig. 4 Different patterns of HMWCK expression identified by antibody 34βE12 in prostatic tissue. (A) Strong expression in basal cells of non-neoplastic glands (upper). Expression is absent from adjacent neoplastic glands in which no basal cells can be identified. Luminal cells contain larger vesicular nuclei. The appearances are subtle and not readily apparent in H&E sections. (B,C) Normal glands with basal cells adjacent to neoplastic glands expressing a diffuse granular cytoplasmic product. In both examples, this pattern is anomalous and does not indicate the presence of basal cells. Focal absence of basal cells indicates those glands in early transition to malignancy. (D) Clearly neoplastic glands in which staining is granular throughout luminal cells and in which no basal cells can be identified morphologically. This is also a pre-malignant variant of 34βE12 expression.

cells,[30] monoclonal antibody clone 34βE12 (known in earlier literature as CK903, EAB903 or hP34) to HMWCKs quickly became used to demonstrate the absence of basal cells from prostatic lesions and hence discriminate between early prostatic malignancy and atypical but non-neoplastic mimics of carcinoma.[31]

On prostatic needle biopsy, atypical glands with a negative HMWCK immunostain, indicating lack of a basal cell layer, are characteristic of prostate cancer (Fig. 4). However, in certain cases, absence of staining from a small focus of atypical glands remains unconvincing and insufficient to make a diagnosis of cancer. Negative HMWCK immunostaining of a small focus of atypical glands is not associated with an increased prediction of prostate cancer on follow-up biopsy (~43%) when compared with previously published data for 'small focus of atypical glands' alone (~45%). Since 48% of men with an initial negative biopsy and multiple follow-up biopsy procedures are found to have cancer, more than one repeat biopsy, or more extensive sampling on the first repeat biopsy, may be necessary to maximise identification of cancer. These findings are comparable with men found with an atypical diagnosis, but without a negative HMWCK immunostain.[32]

As with other monoclonal antibodies, it is important to employ the correct protocol for identifying expression of HMWCKs. In a comparative study of basal cell detection, enzyme pre-digestion and microwave antigen retrieval were found not to yield identical information and that, as a procedural standard, detection of HMWCKs with antibody clone 34βE12 should be employed only after use of a defined microwave-retrieval protocol, when it becomes an extremely sensitive positive marker for high-grade invasive urothelial carcinoma.[33]

Distinction of basal cell hyperplasia (BCH) from carcinoma or high-grade prostatic intraepithelial neoplasia (HGPIN) may be difficult.[1,29] In this situation, use of HMWCK immunostaining can be of crucial assistance. In cribriform BCH, many glands within a focus appear as fused individual BCH glands whereas cribriform prostatic PIN and cribriform cancer glands represent a single glandular unit with a punched-out lumen. In cribriform BCH, HMWCK expression is revealed as a continuous and frequently multilayered staining basal cells in some glands. Conversely, cribriform PIN appears as an interrupted immunoreactive single-cell layer of basal cells. Recognition of the architectural and cytological features of unusual morphologies of BCH can be used to facilitate diagnosis and hence differentiation between prostatic carcinoma and high-grade PIN neoplasia.[34]

α-METHYLACYL-COA-RACEMASE (AMACR)

The gene for α-methylacyl-CoA-racemase (AMACR; also known as P504S, or RACE) maps on chromosome 5, at 5p13.2. It encodes a set of AMACR family members of mitochondrial and peroxisomal enzymes essential in lipid metabolism. Originally identified as a potential discriminator of malignant from benign prostatic epithelium by DNA subtractive hybridisation and microarray techniques,[35] expression of AMACR detected by immuno-histochemistry has been suggested as a molecular marker of prostate cancer detected by needle biopsy.[36-40]

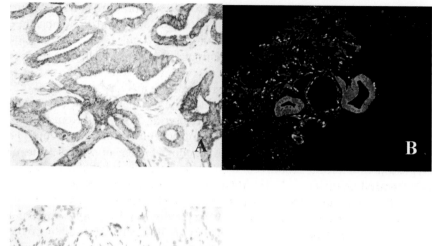

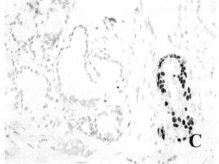

Fig. 5 Cytoplasmic expression of α-methyl Co-A racemase by antibody P504S.
(A) Clearly depicting pre-malignant glandular epithelium with small foci of intervening invasive carcinoma. (B) Immunofluorescence for P504S can be used as a rapid screening technique to localise areas of particular interest. (C) Nuclear localisation of protein p63 independently identify potentially malignant glands. Combined with P504S, this forms a powerful diagnostic cocktail.

An alternatively spliced form (AMACR IIA) differs from AMACR IA by having an alternative exon 5, and is expressed 5–10 times less abundantly.[41] A further three variants have been described, and designated as IB, IIB and IIAs.[42] In contrast to AMACR IA, variants IIA, IIAs, IB and IIB are basic proteins that lack the PTS1 peptide. In prostate tissues that overexpress AMACR, the A and the B forms are both overexpressed, suggesting possible co-regulation. However, specific difference in localisation and function of the variants are yet to be elucidated.

Immunocytochemical staining with antibodies to AMACR exhibits strong reactivity in the majority of prostatic carcinomas (Fig. 5), while normal and benign prostatic epithelium remains unstained, or stained only weakly and/or focally.[35,43–45] In contrast to HMWCKs which are 'negative' basal cell markers, AMACR is a 'positive' marker, its expression being enhanced in prostate cancer cells, and is thus potentially more useful as a diagnostic tool. Since negative absence of staining by basal cell markers, especially in small foci of atypical glands, is not necessarily diagnostic of prostate cancer, positive staining for AMACR can increase the level of confidence in establishing a definitive diagnosis of malignancy.

Presently, there is only one commercial source for an antibody against AMACR in formalin-fixed paraffin-embedded material and this is a rabbit monoclonal (Zeta Corp., Sierra Madre, CA, USA). However, we have recently had the opportunity to evaluate an alternative antibody (DakoCytomation, Ely, UK), which, according to the protocol developed in our laboratory, shows comparable reactivity (unpublished observations).

Staining for AMACR has its greatest utility in resolving diagnostic uncertainties that arise in prostatic needle biopsies containing small foci of suspicious cells. One study reported a sensitivity for AMACR staining to be 94.5%.[37] AMACR immunostaining has also been found to improve diagnostic resolution of such uncertainty beyond that obtained with other immuno-cytochemical markers such as HMWCKs.[39] However, other authors have found that prostate cancer cells present in needle biopsies were positively stained by AMACR in only 80% of cases.[36,38,40] Differences in reported sensitivity are probably due to variations in tissue fixation and immunocyto-chemical methodology.

Another technical consideration is recognition of endogenous biotin staining when avidin–biotin-based detection systems are employed in conjunction with HMAR. In such circumstances appropriate negative control sections (i.e. ones that have been subjected to HMAR in a similar way to test sections) should be carefully scrutinised.[46] This is especially important here, since endogenous biotin and AMACR reaction products have a similar granular appearance, and cytoplasmic distribution pattern. Alternatively, endogenous biotin blockade may be employed, or perhaps preferentially, a non-biotin based detection system such as a labelled-polymer system may be used.

HGPIN is reported as overexpressing AMACR in about two-thirds of cases.[47] Benign glands may stain, albeit weakly and/or focally, in between 16%[37] and 21%[36] of cases. Two uncommon variants of prostate cancer that often pose diagnostic challenges on needle biopsy are the foamy gland and pseudohypoplastic carcinomas. In this setting, application of AMACR immunohistochemistry can provide a valuable diagnostic adjunct. When a pathologist diagnoses one of these variants on routine H+E stained sections, and stains for basal cells are negative, yet a definitive diagnosis of cancer remains difficult because of the cancer's deceptively benign appearance, then a positive staining for AMACR can provide additional confidence to establish a definitive malignant diagnosis. However, the major caveat in the interpretation of positive staining is that high-grade PIN cannot be part of the differential diagnosis.[48]

An elevated level of AMACR expression is not restricted to cases of prostatic neoplasia. Strong positive immunocytochemical staining in proximal tubules and glomerular epithelial cells of the kidney, and in hepatocytes, with several other normal cell types staining moderately or weakly has been reported.[44] Additionally, AMACR staining may have utility in tumours other than those arising from prostatic epithelium. In renal cell carcinomas, strong immunocytochemical staining has been reported in 100% of papillary renal cell carcinomas, but only focal and/or weak reactivity in 15% (18/124) of other renal tumours.[49] Hence, AMACR does not have utility as an indicator of the primary site in cases of metastatic disease. An interesting corollary to the use of AMACR in diagnosis is the suggestion that elevated levels of AMACR activity may be specifically detected in needle biopsies by real-time analysis in the clinic.[50]

Successful management of early prostate cancer either by radical surgery followed by irradiation or by irradiation alone (external beam or brachytherapy), and the treatment of urinary bladder cancer by radiotherapy, has resulted in increasing numbers of requests for pathologists to identify post-irradiation prostate cancer. Morphologically, this can be extremely difficult due to the altered micro-anatomic relationships between cells in an irradiated field as well as the altered cytomorphology of individual cells (epithelial and stromal) as a consequence of the irradiation. In this setting, AMACR has been shown to be a highly specific and sensitive indicator of post-irradiation prostate cancer, discriminating between benign and malignant prostatic glands of altered morphology.[51]

p63 EXPRESSION

p63 is a p53-homologue consistently expressed by basal cells of stratified epithelia, including myoepithelial cells of the breast and basal cells of the prostate.[52] The gene for p63 is located on chromosome 3q27 and encodes six isoforms. While the three transactivating isoforms may act as tumour suppressor genes, the DeltaN-isoforms may inhibit the p53/TA-p63-driven cell-cycle arrest and apoptosis pathway.[53] Distinction between different p63 isoforms by mRNA expression in different normal human tissues has been shown to be of fundamental importance when interpreting the biological phenotype of cells containing the identified protein.[54] A shift in balance between different p63 isoforms promotes or inhibits normal or malignant growth, depending upon simultaneous co-expression of other co-acting genes. In contrast to the tumour-suppressor function of p53, overexpression of select p63 splice variants is observed in many carcinomas (Fig. 5C) supporting the concept that p63 acts as an oncogene.[55]

Unlike p53, whose protein expression is not readily detectable in epithelial cells unless exposed to various conditions of stress (particularly mutation-inducing), p63 is expressed in only select epithelial cells at high levels under normal conditions.

In a comparative assessment of p63 as a potential diagnostic marker of prostatic basal cells, and as a sensitive method of discriminating between prostate cancer and its benign mimics (in comparison with HMWCK identified by 34βE12), no case revealed discordance between identification by the two markers. In the control arm of the study, no false-positive staining was identified while there was less false-negative staining for p63 when compared with that of HMWCK. It was concluded that p63 staining, alone, is at least as sensitive and specific for identification of prostatic basal cells as 34βE12.[56] Unfortunately, this and other studies[57] were performed before the existence and biological relevance of p63 isoforms were understood. Such considerations emphasise the necessity to know the genetic location of the encoded epitope identified by a particular monoclonal antibody before the biological relevance of a particular staining pattern can be interpreted in a biologically meaningful manner.

BASAL CELL-SPECIFIC COCKTAILS

The difficulty with prostatic needle biopsies arises not only from the small amount of tissue available for histological examination but also because biopsies often identify only a few glands which may be either malignant or one of several histological benign mimics of cancer. In some cases, particularly with small foci, an ambiguous lesion may be cut-out in subsequent adjacent slides required for immunohistochemistry. Qualitative differences have been identified between 34βE12 and p63 in the patterns of staining prostatic tissues, these have been found to be clinically significant in situations where p63 staining offered diagnostic utility beyond that of 34βE12.[58] In such cases, p63 staining appeared as strong but discontinuous in atypical glands and adjacent benign glands whereas 34βE12 failed to stain optimally these structures, thus emphasising the necessity for the accurate use of a standard defined protocol for immunostaining.[59] To avoid such difficulties, various cocktails of antibodies have been suggested. Association of an antibody which detects AMACR (p5045) with one which detects p63 as a useful marker of neoplastic transformation in the prostate gland has demonstrated increased sensitivity up to 97% and specificity of up to 100% on routine biopsy specimens. This combination of antibodies identifies basal cell layers more intensely than either 34βE12 or p63 alone and has a staining pattern identical to that of 34βE12. However, immunohistochemistry of prostatic glands from the transition zone is subject to staining variability that results in frequent variable and occasional negative basal cell staining in histologically benign glands. While 34βE12 is prone to such variability, the basal cell cocktail is least susceptible to such variation and not only increases sensitivity of basal cell detection but also reduces staining variability and enhances consistencies of basal cell immunostaining. Additional support for such a combination has been provided by the anecdotal findings that the combined use of p504S as a positive marker and p63 as a negative marker allows for reduction in false/negative interpretation, improved sensitivity and specificity, fewer slides required reduced technical time and the percentage of ambiguous lesions and the necessity for a further biopsy.[60,61]

An alternate cocktail of antibodies to p63, cytokeratins 5/6 and cytokeratin 14, was found to be of value in detecting basal cells in the presence of poorly-differentiated carcinomas, or carcinomas of unknown origin, while individual use of any of these three markers failed to identify the cells detected by the combination.[62]

In cases of small foci, ambiguous lesions might disappear and certainly change in morphological appearance, between the two adjacent tissue sections. Therefore, studies have been performed to combine two or more antibodies and hence assist detection of malignant cells, particularly resolving continued uncertainty over the malignant potential of HGPIN or AAH. These have suggested that combined p63/p504S immunostaining is a sensitive and specific detector of prostatic adenocarcinoma and HGPIN and is thus useful if the evaluation of atypical acini suspicious for adenocarcinoma.[44,63,64]

IDENTIFICATION OF GENOTYPIC SUBTYPES OF PROSTATE CANCER

In an individual biopsy, identification of a group of abnormal prostatic epithelial cells to contain an identifiable genetic mutation is a powerful adjunct for making the diagnosis of prostate cancer. Antibodies to tumour suppressor genes p53 and pRb are commonly employed in many histopathology laboratories and, therefore, are available for such purpose. When applying these reagents, distinction should be drawn between those specifically prostate-associated and those that identify a process that is likely to be cancer-related. Provided that the investigator understands the value of each type of reagent, and employs each in an appropriate manner, then the derived information can be extremely valuable in each individual instance.

p53 TUMOUR SUPPRESSOR GENE

Mutation in the p53 gene occurs in about 40% of prostate cancers. It is current dogma that some mutations in the expressed protein result in a non-functional protein that is retained at high and easily detectable levels within the nucleus or cytoplasm of affected cells. Assuming this to be correct, then the presence of p53-positive cells within a prostate biopsy, particularly those containing an identifiable micro-anatomic lesion, confirms the presence of an important genetic mutation. Given that such staining patterns are the consequence of a

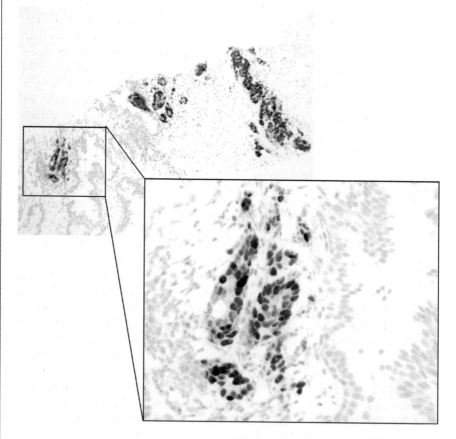

Fig. 6 While not confirming malignancy, mutated p53 defines potentially malignant epithelia that may initially appear morphologically unremarkable. The glandular distribution of p53 expression and the cytomorphological features revealed on close inspection confirm the probably malignant nature of these glands.

mutational event, and not the consequence of some non-neoplastic event such as inflammation or sclerosing adenosis, then the effect is to focus attention on specific regions of the biopsy (Fig. 6).

Pathologists should be aware that although p53 staining identifies a genetic mutation, it does not *ipso facto*, confirm the presence of prostate cancer, although its presence is an extremely powerful adjunct. The protein product(s) of the p53 gene is/are extremely important and powerful regulators of cellular behaviour. Not only is p53 one of the signal tumour-suppressor genes within all cells, but it also exerts important regulatory control on apoptosis[65] and androgen receptor-mediated signalling.[66]

PRB TUMOUR SUPPRESSOR GENE

Tumour suppressor gene pRb located on chromosome 7q21 is associated early with the development of prostate cancer in a minority of cases. In contrast to p53, mutation of the pRb genome results in non-expression of the protein products of this gene, in stark contrast to its strong nuclear expression in the nuclei of all surrounding cells. In a similar manner to p53, whilst not confirming prostate cancer, absence of pRb staining from a particular micro-anatomic appearance is strong adjunctive evidence for malignant transformation of those particular epithelial cells. Presently, genetic evidence does not form part of the compendium of criteria with which to make the diagnosis of prostate cancer or to distinguish between 'severe dysplasia', 'PIN' and 'carcinoma *in situ*'. While the morphological criteria are currently the gold standard by which these entities are diagnosed, the use of antibodies to p53 and to pRb provide valuable objective evidence of an important genetic change, thus providing impartial evidence to support the diagnosis of 'cancer' rather than 'dysplasia'.

BCL-2

Overexpression of apoptosis-suppressing oncoproteins results in defective apoptotic signalling and is probably a common occurrence in prostate cancer.[67] Inhibition of apoptosis or disruption of cell death signalling promotes carcinogenesis and may play a role in cancer initiation.[68,69] Early studies of the Bcl-2 gene revealed an intricate relationship between cell death disruption and carcinogenesis.[70,71] This genetic alteration causes overexpression of Bcl-2 and concomitant down-regulation of cell death. Since the discovery of Bcl-2, at least six other homologues have been identified, including Bax, bcl-X, Bad, and Bak. Additional forms arise through alternative splicing.[72] These exist as intracellular proteins, predominantly found in the outer mitochondrial membrane, nuclear envelope and endoplasmic reticulum.[73] Overexpression of the protein in cancer cells may block or delay onset of apoptosis, selecting and maintaining long-living cells, and arresting cells in the G_0 phase of the cell cycle.[74,75] Bcl-2 protects against a wide variety of cell death signals, and probably does so by controlling signalling.[76,77]

Expression of Bcl-2 is usually restricted to the basal cell layer of the non-neoplastic and hyperplastic (Fig. 7) prostatic epithelium.[78] However, overexpression of Bcl-2 is present in PIN.[79,80] In prostate cancer, the prevalence

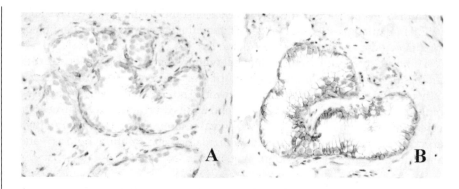

Fig. 7 (A) Bcl-2. In normal prostate glands, this protein is strongly expressed by basal cells. In atypical (but benign) epithelial hyperplasia, this protein can be expressed cytoplasmically throughout the hyperplastic compartment. In malignancy, Bcl-2 expression is lost early, although cells resembling basal cells may remain. (B) HER-2/*neu*. Presence of this protein is the reciprocal of Bcl-2 in that *de novo* expression appears early extending throughout the neoplastic compartment, irrespective of morphology. Hence, the combination of p53 (or p63) together with loss of Bcl-2 and gain of HER-2/*neu* are powerful immunohistochemical discriminators of prostatic malignancy.

and expression pattern of Bcl-2 are controversial. One study found moderate heterogeneous Bcl-2 overexpression in localised cancer,[79,80] which was inversely correlated with Gleason grade. Another report described a significant elevation of Bcl-2 in 45% of cases of primary cancer, which was heterogeneous but did not correlate with grade. Metastatic cancer in lymph nodes was negative. Another study found over 70% of prostate carcinomas to be Bcl-2 negative, 18% had weak expression, and 11% exhibited strong expression.[81] Expression of Bcl-2 was correlated with high stage, high grade and presence of metastases. Androgen deprivation therapy decreased Bcl-2 in cancer, suggesting that these cells develop resistance to apoptotic signals.[82–84] In hormone-refractory prostate cancer, heterogeneous staining was observed in most specimens, with expression retained in clusters of cancer cells. In bone marrow metastases after androgen deprivation, Bcl-2 was present in about 30% of cancers although expression did not correlate with survival.[85] In summary, reports of Bcl-2 expression in prostate cancer vary greatly. The data support the concept that Bcl-2 is causally linked to apoptotic resistance in prostatic cancer cells.

HER2/*neu*

HER2/*neu* is a glycoprotein that has homology with the epidermal growth factor receptor and has been implicated in the malignant transformation and tumourigenesis of a variety of epithelia, although best analysed in breast.[86,87] Encoded in a gene located on chromosome 17q 11.2-q12, there are potentially 22 protein isoforms whose expression is controlled by at least 9 alternate promoters. Using a polyclonal antibody (DakoCytomation, UK) Her2/*neu* is not expressed by non-neoplastic cells but appears at a low level as neoplasia develops and appreciably enhances as malignancy becomes established. This relationship appears to be quantitatively reciprocal to the expression of Bcl-2 (Fig. 7), as in the breast and bladder. Furthermore, there is some evidence that Her2/*neu* expression in prostate carcinoma varies by clinical state such that HER2/*neu* expression can be defined within individual patients, as their disease progresses.[88] It has been suggested that HER2/*neu* is overexpressed in 25% of untreated prostate carcinoma specimens, in 59% of specimens treated with hormones before surgery, in 78% of patients with androgen-independent disease[89] and in 80% of metastasis disease cases.[90] Thus, HER2/*neu* immunohistochemistry may provide objective information on the early development of neoplasia and or of assisting the diagnosis of malignancy. In the latter, it may be that expression of individual splice variants can assist in prediction of the likely behavioural or response-status of the identified prostate cancer.

PREDICTION OF THE BEHAVIOURAL PHENOTYPE OF PROSTATE CANCER

HEAT SHOCK PROTEINS

Heat shock proteins are normal cellular proteins expressed under non-stressed conditions in a cell cycle-dependent manner.[91,92] Some are chaperonins of nascent proteins and have defined roles as regulators of protein homeostasis under both normal and cytologically adverse conditions.[93] In neoplasia, heat shock proteins have been implicated in multidrug resistance,[183] in regulating apoptosis[94] and as modulators of p53 activity.[95] hsp-27 is a member of the low-molecular-weight family and constitutively expressed at low levels in the cytosol of most human cells.[96] In early prostatic neoplasia, normal expression of hsp-27 appears to be down-regulated prior to development of invasive malignancy such that its absence draws attention to those regions that are involved in early stages of neoplasia (Fig. 7). However, following invasion of adjacent stromal connective tissues, expression of hsp-27 may be modulated such that it either remains down-regulated or its expression becomes enhanced. The level of expression correlates with aggressiveness of the individual prostate cancer[97] and is thus a potentially valuable marker of the behavioural phenotype. In the problematic prostatic biopsy, absence of hsp-27 expression signifies areas of concern, particularly foci of probable malignant transformation, since down-regulation of this marker does not appear to be mediated by non-neoplastic events, including inflammation. Conversely, renewed expression in an invasive prostatic malignancy specifies an aggressive phenotype.

PROTEIN KINASE C ISOENZYMES

Protein kinase C (PKC) isoenzymes are serine/threonine kinases that play major roles in transmembrane signal transduction pathways. Some have functions in pathways that are in common with hsp-27, co-regulating expression of oestrogen receptors within prostatic epithelial cells. Thus, it is not surprising that the expression of PKC-β appears to be modulated in a manner similar to hsp-27 during early prostatic neoplasia and genesis of the

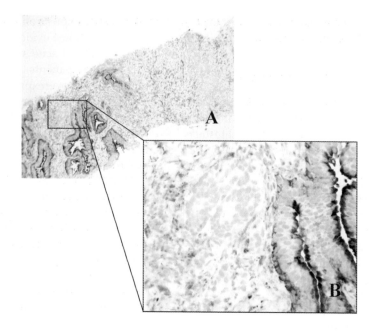

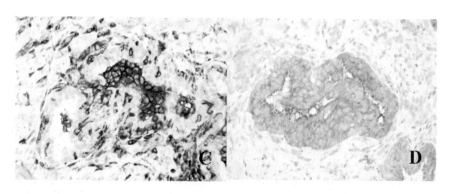

Fig. 8 Combination of heat shock proteins and protein kinase C isoenzymes also identify the malignant phenotype that may not be apparent morphologicaly. (A,B) Loss of normal hsp-27 expression is recognised as a neoplastic (possibly pre-malignant)event. (C) Loss of PCK-β from intraglandular epithelium may be accompanied by its re-expression in the adjacent invasive carcinoma cells where it signifies poor prognosis. (D) *De novo* expression of PKC-ζ defines those prostatic epithelial cells that are developing invasive phenotype, and are hence potentially pre-malignant.

malignant phenotype. Loss of PKC-β staining is a sensitive indicator of regions of *in situ* neoplasia and a predictor of the likely behavioural phenotype.[98]

In contrast, PKC-ζ is not expressed by non-neoplastic prostatic epithelium but appears only in the malignant phenotype (Fig. 8). While a potentially powerful marker of invasive malignancy, its expression appears inconsistent such that it might identify only a subset of invasive carcinomas which, unlike E2F3, hsp-27 or PKC-β, have not yet been confirmed to correlate with aggressive behaviour. Expression of PKC-ζ is governed by two potential promoters and may occur as any of seven splice-variant proteins. It is likely that this inconsistency is determined by the splice variant of PKC-ζ and the particular promoter region.

ION CHANNEL EXPRESSION

To become invasive and metastatic, prostate cancer cells require the expression of functional Na+ channels of a type previously only identified in electrically-active tissues such as nerve and muscle.[99] Work on human prostate carcinoma cell lines confirmed broadly comparable properties of ion channels expressed *de novo* when compared to other tissues. More extensive studies found a strong correlation between Na+ channel expression in prostate cancer lines and their invasiveness *in vitro*.[100,101] Differential expression of voltage-gated Na+ and K+ (and possibly other) channels in prostate cancer cells of varying metastatic potential, and demonstration of their function in cellular behaviour (such as proliferation and invasion), are consistent with voltage-gated ion channels having a significant role in the metastatic process. This complements other findings showing that ion channel expression is altered during cancer progression.[99,100] Thus, ion channels may represent novel markers of metastasis in prostate and hence form part of the definition of the metastatic malignant phenotype.

MICROVESSEL DENSITY AND PREDICTION OF PATHOLOGICAL STAGE

Microvessel density (MVD) analysis offers promise for predicting pathological stage and patient outcome in prostate cancer. The microvessels associated with prostate cancer are shorter than those in benign or hyperplastic prostatic tissue, with more undulating vessel walls.[102,103] Cumulative evidence suggests an important role for MVD analysis in managing select patients with prostate cancer. Different authors have employed various reagents to detect endothelial cells and hence activate microvessel density. None of these antigenic or epitopic determinants are endothelium-specific. Furthermore, due to phenotypic heterogeneity, none identified all endothelial cells. The most commonly employed antibodies are to blood-coagulation Factor VIII, while the lectin to *Ulex europaeus* specifically recognised oligosaccharide structure fucose α1→3 expressed to high levels on newly-formed vascular (including lymphatic) channels.

A range of different studies have investigated the relationship of MVD and prostate cancer stage.[104–115] While most compared MVD in prostatectomy specimens with pathological stage, two assessed MVD in contemporary needle biopsies and correlated it with pathological stage at prostatectomy.[113,114] Two others compared MVD in transurethral resections from patients undergoing irradiation[108] or predominantly watchful waiting[109] with clinical stage. On prostatic biopsy, MVD in cancer showed a positive correlation with matched prostatectomies and was an independent predictor of extraprostatic extension.[113,114] When optimised MVD was added to Gleason score and serum PSA concentration, the predictive value of these measures for stage increased significantly. There is generally good agreement about prediction of cancer recurrence based on MVD[108,109,116,117] and microvascular invasion[116] predicted biochemical (PSA) failure. When most patients were treated only with palliative hormonal manipulation, MVD did not predict progression independent of grade.[109] MVD did not correlate with biochemical failure after controlling for stage (pT2) and grade (Gleason grade 6 and higher) in patients treated by radical prostatectomy.[117] Three studies addressed the potential of MVD[109,118] or microvascular invasion[119] to predict cancer-specific survival, and found no independent predictive value. The predictive value on univariate analysis was negated by inclusion of grade[109,119] or stage.[118]

p9KA

Protein p9Ka is a strictly intracellular molecule belonging to the S100 class of Ca^{2+}-binding molecules. Direct correlation has been confirmed between expression of p9Ka mRNA and protein with the metastatic phenotype of prostate cancer cells.[120] Immunofluorescence studies have indicated that recombinant p9Ka binds to specific sites on at least two intracellular polypeptides and that it is located on cytoskeletal components in a pattern identical with the distribution of actin filaments.[121] The primary function of p9Ka appears to be a molecular organiser specifically activated by differential Ca^{2+} binding. Immunohistochemical studies of human prostate cancer using novel monoclonal antibodies to p9Ka peptides confirm enhanced expression of this protein in metastatic cells.

MITOTIC AND APOPTOTIC MARKERS

Mitotic figures

Mitotic figures are rarely found in tissue sections in normal or hyperplastic prostatic epithelium. Therefore, S-phase markers are commonly used as surrogates for estimating proliferation rates. Cells in the DNA synthetic phase of the cell cycle incorporate the thymidine analogue bromodeoxyuridine (BRdU) into newly synthesised DNA and also express both proliferative cell nuclear antigen (PCNA)[122] and Ki-67 antigens.[123] One study of BRdU, PCNA, and Ki-67 labelling in prostatic tissues demonstrated that the three methods are strongly correlated with each other.[124] The number of mitotic figures increased progressively from benign epithelium through PIN to cancer.[124–128] Adenocarcinomas with cribriform growth pattern and those composed of solid areas of undifferentiated tumour cells contained most mitotic figures.[129] The number of mitotic figures correlated with cancer stage and grade,[124,127,130–133] as well as with progression and progression-free survival.[132] Androgen deprivation therapy results in a dramatic decline in the number of mitotic figures in prostate cancer,[127,134] whereas normal prostatic epithelium undergoes apoptosis-mediated involution.[135] Thus, it appears that elevation in epithelial cell proliferation parallels cancer progression and that determinants of elevated cellular proliferation have significant potential value as prognostic markers.

Ki-67 expression

Ki-67 is a non-histone nuclear protein expressed by proliferating cells in the G_0 phase of the cell cycle. Since the original antibodies to Ki-67 exhibited only

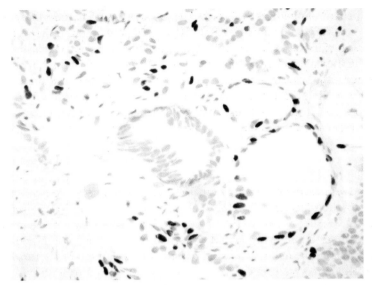

Fig. 9 It is incorrect to presume that elevated proliferation, as determined by Ki-67 staining defines the malignant component of a tissue. Proliferation and invasion are biologically different such that, in prostatic biopsy diagnostic practice, proliferation markers do not contribute to the identification of prostate cancer.

poor immunoreactivity in fixed paraffin-embedded tissues, the MIB-1 monoclonal antibody was developed against recombinant parts of the Ki-67 antigen for specific use on formalin-fixed and paraffin wax-embedded tissues.[184] Originally, it was suggested that Ki-67 labelling indices correlated with cancer.[136,137] However, in prostate cancer, a high proliferation index (Fig. 9) identified within the MIB-1 antibody appears to add little predictive information for patient outcome above the traditional indicators of Gleason score, pathological stage, and DNA ploidy.[138] However, the Ki-67 labelling index may discriminate between organ-confined and metastatic cancer.[124] Hence, elevation in Ki-67 proliferation indices appear to reflect progression.[139,140] This is further reflected in an association between expression of Ki-67 and the EGFR,[185] mutant p53,[141,142] particular chromosomal aberrations,[143] and perineural invasion.[144] Taken together, all of these findings suggested that Ki-67 expression may be a weak prognostic indicator of recurrence,[145,146] progression,[140,147] and survival.[142,146,148] Studies by McLoughlin et al.,[149] Feneley et al.,[150] and Speights et al.[151] all confirm that Ki-67 identification using the MIB-1 antibody does not predict clinical outcome, except in the very worst prognosis cases. However, in post-radiation recurrence prostatic adenocarcinoma, the sole proliferation index by MIB-1 reached independent significance. Diagnostically, this may become an important diagnostic factor as the numbers of patients surviving long-term following radical radiotherapy increases.[152]

Apoptotic markers

Apoptotic bodies are present throughout all normal prostatic epithelia. Usually present in intercellular spaces, but occasionally within the cytoplasm of epithelial cells, the latter being observed more often in PIN and carcinoma than in benign epithelium.[153] In non-neoplastic prostatic tissues, the greatest frequency is invariably in the basal cell layer. In carcinoma, the apoptotic process occurs in cells at the periphery of the malignant glands adjacent to the stroma. Detectable by activated caspase-3 immunohistochemistry, the percentage of apoptotic bodies has been estimated to be progressively higher in low-grade PIN, high-grade PIN, and adenocarcinoma than in BPH (0.68%, 0.75%, and 0.92% to 2.10% versus 0.26%, respectively) but with no apparent correlation between the numbers of mitotic figures and apoptotic bodies.

Derangement of apoptosis appears to play a critical role in the pathogenesis of prostate cancer.[67,83,154,155] There is down-regulation of apoptotic rates and up-regulation of proliferative indices in localised prostatic cancer when compared with adjacent normal tissues.[80] Cell proliferation rates were higher than apoptotic rates, resulting in a net gain in cell number in localised and metastatic carcinoma. The apoptotic rate of an individual prostatic carcinoma provided more accurate prognostic information than the proliferation rate. There was a significant elevation in apoptotic count in high-grade cancer and those with aggressive progression profiles.[67,84,156–158] Cancer with perineural invasion had a lower apoptotic rate than that with invasion,[159] perhaps accounting for the frequent tumour spread through perineural spaces.[160] The molecular mechanisms underlying a lower apoptotic rate in carcinomas with perineural invasion appeared not to be due to overexpression of Bcl-2[161] but to an unidentified nerve-derived factor(s) because the apoptotic rates were negatively correlated with the diameter of the nerves. This finding suggests that micro-environment influences apoptotic activity, and hence the growth potential of carcinomas, which, in turn, controls tumour progression and metastasis. Androgen-deprivation therapy increased the apoptotic rate in prostate cancer.[84,127,162]

NEUROENDOCRINE MARKERS

Neuroendocrine cells are part of the widely dispersed diffuse neuroendocrine regulatory system, also known as endocrine–paracrine cells. In the human prostate, subpopulations of neuroendocrine cells have been identified based on morphology and secretory products.[163] Most neuroendocrine cells of the prostate contain serotonin,[164] chromogranin A,[165] bombesin[166] and other neuroendocrine markers that are not consistently expressed. Based on their function in other organs, neuroendocrine cells in the prostate are probably involved in regulation of growth, differentiation, and secretory functions. In human prostatic carcinoma, neuroendocrine differentiation appears as: (i) infrequent small cell neuroendocrine carcinoma; (ii) rare carcinoid-like cancer; and (iii) conventional prostatic cancer with focal neuroendocrine differentiation.[167] Proponents of a role for neuroendocrine differentiation have shown that the neuroendocrine cell population enlarges with cancer progression,[168] appears to correlate with Gleason sum and cancer stage,[169] could be a prognostic factor for progression,[169–171] and elevated serum levels of chromogranin A may detect prostate cancer in patients whose PSA is not elevated.[165,172] Conversely, the detractors for a role of neuroendocrine differentiation have shown that the neuroendocrine cell population does not exhibit any relationship with cell proliferation,[140] is not associated with pathological stage or Gleason sum[140,173] or other measures of progression[173] such as increasing serum PSA,[174] is not correlated with cancer-specific survival,[175] and, therefore, has no independent prognostic significance for prostate cancer.[173,175,176] Since neuroendocrine cells lack androgen receptors,[167] there is no alteration in the extent of neuroendocrine cell differentiation following hormonal manipulation.[167]

ANDROGEN RECEPTOR GENE

Androgen-receptor (AR) gene mutations are present in prostate cancer before hormonal therapy and in hormone-refractory cancer. Activation of mutant AR by oestrogen and weak androgens may confer on cancer cells an ability to survive testicular androgen deprivation by allowing activation of the AR by adrenal androgens or exogenous oestrogen.[166] Such mutations might confer a growth advantage even without androgen deprivation because prostate cancer has lower levels of 5-AR and DHT than normal tissue.[177]

Androgen activity depends largely on the presence of androgen-binding components or 'receptors' which are present in the nucleus of prostatic epithelial basal, stromal cells and possibly differentiated neuroendocrine cells. Studies of AR in prostate carcinoma have often been contradictory, and currently there is no consensus on the usefulness of AR staining in prostate carcinoma. AR staining does not necessarily reflect a structurally intact, functionally, active receptor. Correlations of staining with grade have been noted by some, but not by others.[178] One study showed greater variability in AR staining in tumours with poor response to androgen ablation.[179] Another showed no correlation between staining and time to progression of disease.[139] Finally, a recent study employing image analysis techniques showed that mean concentration of AR in tumour cells is the principal predictor of outcome in patients undergoing hormonal ablation therapy for stage D2 diseases.[180]

CONCLUSIONS

Immunohistochemistry provides an increasingly important adjunct to the accurate morphological diagnosis and predictive analysis of prostatic biopsy specimens. Applications range from discrimination of problematic diagnostic appearances to the identification of phenotypically-defined subsets within prostate cancer. These might be aggressive behavioural phenotypes[97,98,101,181] or androgen status or likely response to particular pharmacological therapy.[101,182] However, immunohistochemistry, particularly of small biopsies where a contentious lesion might be cut-through in a few serial tissue-sections, is not facile but requires the judicious use of appropriate reagents in order to answer a defined diagnostic question. Up-coming information from the Human Genome Database has revealed factors such as differential splice variants and gene-truncation at the 5′ or 3′ ends of cancer-expressed proteins to be important considerations with respect to the generation and use of monoclonal antibodies to particular proteins, if erroneous data are not to be generated.

For monoclonal antibodies to be truly valuable, it is essential that commercial companies now provide detailed information with respect to the epitopic location of their individual antibodies. This information should include the type of epitope (*e.g.* whether a primary amino acid sequence or a tertiary structure), and the particular exon being transcribed to contain the epitope. Knowledge of gene expression has progressed to a level of sophistication that this information is required to make a detailed evaluation of the biological and pathological significance of the expression, or loss, of particular genetic regions as well as the factors affecting the identified expression status.

Biomolecular genetic analysis offers an attractive alternative to morphological methods of tissue diagnosis. However, there are many significant constraints to be overcome before a conceptual shift in diagnostic methodology takes place. Nevertheless, there is no doubt that a deep understanding of molecular genetics, not only for the diagnosis of cancer specimens but also for non-malignant conditions of the prostate, will be required by diagnostic surgical pathologists of the near future. Therefore, it would behove those embarking upon a career in diagnostic pathology to begin to understand, and to employ some of the genetic complexities emerging from molecular genetic analysis of human tissues. This information will be required to make diagnoses and to provide appropriate therapies for many different types of patient. Until that time, however, the gold standard will remain high-quality thin-section histomorphology supported by appropriate high-quality immunohistochemistry employed judiciously to answer specific diagnostic questions.

References

1. Foster CS, Sakr WA. Proliferative lesions of the prostate that mimic carcinoma. *Curr Diagn Pathol* 2001; **7:** 194–212.
2. Sternberger LA. *Immunocytochemistry*. Edinburgh: Churchill Livingstone, 1988.
3. Polak JM, Van Noorden S. *Introduction to Immunocytochemistry*. BIOS Scientific, 2002.
4. Kohler G, Milstein C. Continuous culture of fused cells secreting antibody of predefined specificity. *Nature* 1975; **256:** 495–497.
5. Foster C, Gosden CM. HER2/*neu* expression in cancer: the pathologist as diagnostician or prophet? *Hum Pathol* 2003; **34:** 635–638.
6. Foster CS, Edwards PAW, Dinsdale EA, Neville AM. Monoclonal antibodies to the human mammary gland: I. Distribution of determinants in non-neoplastic mammary and extra mammary tissues. *Virol Arch* 1982; **394:** 279–293.
7. Brandtzaeg P. Tissue preparation for immunohistochemistry. In: Bullock P. (ed) *Techniques in Immunohistochemistry*. London: Academic Press, 1982; 1–75.
8. Williams JH, Mepham BL, Wright DH. Tissue preparation for immunocytochemistry. *J Clin Pathol* 1997; **50:** 422–428.
9. Morgan JM, Navabi H, Jasani B. Role of calcium chelation in high temperature antigen retrieval at different pH values. *J Pathol* 1997; **182:** 233–237.
10. Sompuram SR, Vani K, Messana E, Bogen SA. A molecular mechanism of formalin fixation and antigen retrieval. *Am J Clin Pathol* 2004; **121:** 190–199.
11. Huang SN, Minassian H, More JD. Application of immunofluorescent staining on paraffin sections improved by trypsin digestion. *Lab Invest* 1976; **35:** 383–390.
12. Shi SR, Cote C, Kalra KL, Taylor CR, Tandon AK. A technique for retrieving antigens in formalin-fixed, routinely acid-decalcified, celloidin-embedded human temporal bone sections for immunohistochemistry. *J Histochem Cytochem* 1992; **40:** 787–792.
13. Jasani B, Rhodes A. The role and mechanism of high-temperature antigen retrieval in diagnostic pathology. *Curr Diagn Pathol* 2001; **7:** 153–160.

14. Taylor CR, Shi SR, Chen C, Young L, Yang C, Cote RJ. Comparative study of antigen retrieval heating methods: microwave and pressure cooker, autoclave and steamer. *Biotech Histochem* 1996; **71:** 263–270.
15. Pileri SA, Roncador G, Ceccarelli C *et al.* Antigen retrieval techniques in immunohistochemistry: comparison of different methods. *J Pathol* 1997; **183:** 116–123.
16. Shi SR, Cote RJ, Taylor CR. Antigen retrieval techniques: current perspectives. *J Histochem and Cytochem* 2001; **49:** 931–937.
17. Balaton AJ. A systematic approach to quality in immunohistochemistry. *Ann Pathol* 1999; **19:** 299–308.
18. Allsbrook WC, Pfeiffer EA. Histochemistry of the prostate. In: *Major Problems in Pathology.* Philadelphia, PA: W B Saunders, 1998; 282–303.
19. Zhou R, Hammond EH, Sause WT *et al.* Quantitation of prostate-specific acid phosphatase in prostate cancer: reproducibility and correlation with subjective grade. *Modern Pathol* 1994; **7:** 440–448.
20. Kumar A, Goel AS, Hill TM *et al.* Expression of human glandular kallikrein, hK2, in mammalian cells. *Cancer Res* 1996; **56:** 5397–5402.
21. Darson MF, Pacelli A, Roche P *et al.* Human glandular kallikrein 2 (hK2) expression in prostatic intraepithelial neoplasia and adenocarcinoma: a novel prostate cancer marker. *Urology* 1997; **49:** 857–862.
22. Sesterhenn I, Mostofi FK, Davis CJ. Immunopathology of prostate and bladder tumors. In: Russo J. (ed) *Immunocytochemistry in Tumor Diagnosis.* Boston: Martinus Nijhoff, 1985; 337–361.
23. Kishi Y, Kami M, Kusumi E *et al.* Prostatic acid phosphatase (pap): a possible diagnostic marker of intravascular large B-cell lymphoma. *Haematologica* 2004; **89:** ECR13.
24. Mai KT, Collins JP, Veinot JP. Prostatic adenocarcinoma with urotherlial (transitional cell) carcinoma features. *Appl Immunohistochem Mol Morphol* 2002; **10:** 231–236.
25. Weisser H, Krieg M. Kinetic analysis of androstenedione 5 alpha-reductase in epithelium and stroma of human prostate. *Steroids* 1997; **62:** 589–594.
26. Bonkhoff H, Stein U, Aumuller G, Remberger K. Differential expression of 5-alpha-reductase isoenzymes in the human prostate and prostatic carcinomas. *Prostate* 1996; **29:** 261–267.
27. Levine AC, Wang JP, Ren M, Eliashvili E, Russell DW, Kirschenbaum A. Immunohistochemical localization of steroid 5-alpha reductase 2 in the human male fetal reproductive tract and adult prostate. *J Clin Endocrinol Metab* 1996; **81:** 384–394.
28. Bjelfman C, Soderstrom TG, Brekkan E *et al.* Differential gene expression of steroid 5 alpha-reductase 2 in core needle biopsies from malignant and benign prostatic tissue. *J Clin Endocrinol Metab* 1997; **82:** 2210–2214.
29. Foster CS, Sakr W. Exclusion of prostate cancer by pathological assessment of prostatic biopsy specimens. In: Khoury, S, Partin A, Denis L. (eds) *The World Health Organization 5th International Consultation on Benign Prostatic Hyperplasia*, Committee II. Scientific Communication International, 2001; 294–315.
30. Barwick KW, Mardi JA. An immunohistochemical study of the myoepithelial cell in prostate hyperplasia and neoplasia. *Lab Invest* 1983; **48:** 7A.
31. Brawer MK, Peehl DM, Stamey TA, Bostwick DG. Keratin immunoreactivity in the benign and neoplastic human prostate. *Cancer Res* 1985; **45:** 3663–3667.
32. Halushka MK, Kahane H, Epstein JI. Negative 34betaE12 staining in a small focus of atypical glands on prostate needle biopsy: a follow-up study of 332 cases. *Hum Pathol* 2004; **35:** 43–46.
33. Varma M, Morgan M, Amin MB, Wozniak S, Jasani B. High molecular weight cytokeratin antibody (clone 34betaE12): a sensitive marker for differentiation of high-grade invasive urothelial carcinoma from prostate cancer. *Histopathology* 2003; **42:** 167–172.
34. Rioux-Leclercq NC, Epstein JI. Unusual morphological patterns of basal cell hyperplasia of the prostate. *Am J Surg Pathol* 2002; **26:** 237–243.
35. Xu J, Stolk JA, Zhang X *et al.* Identification of differentially expressed genes in human prostate cancer using substraction and microarray. *Cancer Res* 2000; **60:** 1677–1682.
36. Beach R, Gown AM, De Peralta-Venturina MN *et al.* P504S immunohistochemical detection in 405 prostatic specimens including 376 18-gauge needle biopsies. *Am J Surg Pathol* 2002; **26:** 1588–1596.

37. Jiang Z, Wu CL, Woda BA *et al.* P504S/alpha-methylacyl-CoA racemase: a useful marker for diagnosis of small foci of prostatic carcinoma on needle biopsy. *Am J Surg Pathol* 2002; **26**: 1169–1174.

38. Magi-Galluzzi C, Luo J, Isaacs WB, Hicks JL, De Marzo AM, Epstein JI. Alpha-methylacyl-CoA racemase: a variably sensitive immunohistochemical marker for the diagnosis of small prostate cancer foci on needle biopsy. *Am J Surg Pathol* 2003; **27**: 1128–1133.

39. Jiang Z, Iczkowski KA, Woda BA, Tretiakova M, Yang XJ. P504S immunostaining boosts diagnostic resolution of 'suspicious' foci in prostatic needle biopsy specimens. *Am J Clin Pathol* 2004; **121**: 99–107.

40. Zhou M, Aydin H, Kanane H, Epstein JI. How often does alpha-methylacyl-CoA-racemase contribute to resolving an ayptical diagnosis on prostate needle biopsy beyond that provided by basal cell markers? *Am J Surg Pathol* 2004; **28**: 239–243.

41. Shen-Ong GL, Feng DA, Troyer DA. Expression profiling identifies a novel alpha-methylacyl-CoA racemase exon with fumarate hydratase homology. *Cancer Res* 2003; **63**: 3296–3301.

42. Mubiru JN, Shen-Ong GL, Valente AJ, Troyer DA. Alternative spliced variants of the alpha-methylacyl-CoA racemase gene and their expression in prostate cancer. *Gene* 2004; **327**: 89–98.

43. Jiang Z, Woda BA, Rock KL *et al.* P504S: a new molecular marker for the detection of prostate carcinoma. *Am J Surg Pathol* 2001; **25**: 1397–1404.

44. Luo J, Zha S, Gage WR *et al.* Alpha-methylacyl-CoA racemase: a new molecular marker for prostate cancer. *Cancer Res* 2002; **62**: 2220–2226.

45. Rubin MA, Zhou M, Dhanasekaran SM *et al.* Alpha-methylacyl coenzyme A racemase as a tissue biomarker for prostate cancer. *JAMA* 2002; **287**: 1662–1670.

46. Dodson A, Campbell F. Biotin inclusions: a potential pitfall in immunohistochemistry avoided. *Histopathology* 1999; **34**: 178–179.

47. Zhou M, Chinnaiyan AM, Kleer CG, Lucas PC, Rubin MA. Alpha-methylacyl-CoA racemase: a novel tumor marker over-expressed in several human cancers and their precursor lesions. *Am J Surg Pathol* 2002; **26**: 926–931.

48. Zhou M, Jiang Z, Epstein JI. Expression and diagnostic utility of alpha-methylacyl-CoA-racemase (P504S) in foamy gland and pseudohyperplastic prostate cancer. *Am J Surg Pathol* 2003; **27**: 772–778.

49. Tretiakova MS, Sahoo S, Takahashi M *et al.* Expression of alpha-methylacyl-CoA racemase in papillary renal cell carcinoma. *Am J Surg Pathol* 2004; **28**: 69–76.

50. Kumar-Sinha C, Shah RB, Laxman B *et al.* Elevated alpha-methylacyl-CoA racemase enzymatic activity in prostate cancer. *Am J Pathol* 2004; **164**: 787–793.

51. Yang XJ, Laven B, Tretiakova M *et al.* Detection of alpha-methylacyl-coenzyme A racemase in postradiation prostatic adenocarcinoma. *Urology* 2003; **62**: 282–286.

52. Stefanou D, Batistatou A, Nonni A, Arkoumani E, Agnantis NJ. p63 expression in benign and malignant breast lesions. *Histol Histopathol* 2004; **19**: 465–471.

53. Reis-Filho JH, Schmitt FC. Taking advantage of basic research: p63 is a reliable myoepithelial and stem cell marker. *Adv Anat Pathol* 2002; **9**: 280–289.

54. Vincek V, Knowles J, Li J, Nassiri M. Expression of p63 mRNA isoforms in normal human tissue. *Anticancer Res* 2003; **23**: 3945–3948.

55. Westfall MD, Pietenpol JA. p63: Molecular complexity in development and cancer. *Carcinogenesis* 2004; **25**: 857–864.

56. Weinstein MH, Signoretti S, Loda M. Diagnostic utility of immunohistochemical staining for p63, a sensitive marker of prostatic basal cells. *Modern Pathol* 2002; **15**: 1302–1308.

57. Davis LD, Zhang W, Merseburger A *et al.* p63 expression profile in normal and malignant prostate epithelial cells. *Anticancer Res* 2002; **22**: 3819–3825.

58. Shah RB, Zhou M, LeBlanc M, Snyder M, Rubin MA. Comparison of the basal-cell-specific markers, 34betaE12 and p63, in the diagnosis of prostate cancer. *Am J Surg Pathol* 2002; **26**: 1161–1168.

59. Zhou M, Shah R, Shen R, Rubin MA. Basal cell cocktail (34betaE12 + p63) improves the detection of prostate basal cells. *Am J Surg Pathol* 2003; **27**: 365–371.

60. Molinie V, Herve JM, Lugagne PM, Baglin AC. p63 and p504s cocktail is useful in ambiguous lesions of the prostate. *Histopathology* 2004; **44**: 399–408.

61. Tacha DE, Miller RT. Use of p63/P504S monoclonal antibody cocktail in immunohistochemical staining of prostate tissue. *Appl Immunohistochem Mol Morphol* 2004; **12**: 75–78.

62. Reis-Filho JS, Simpson PT, Martins A, Preto A, Gartner F, Schmitt FC. Distribution of p63, cytokeratins 5/6 and cytokeratin 14 in 51 normal and 400 neoplastic human tissue samples using TARP-4 multi-tumor tissue microarray. *Virchows Arch* 2003; **443**: 122–132.

63. Molinie VV, Fromont G, Sibony M *et al.* Diagnostic utility of a p63/alpha-methyl-CoA-racemase (p504s) cocktail in atypical foci in the prostate. *Modern Pathol* 2004; **17**: 1180–1190.

64. Sanderson SO, Sebo TJ, Murphy LM, Neumann R, Slezak J, Cheville JC. An analysis of the p63/alpha-methylacyl coenzyme A racemase immunohistochemical cocktail stain in prostate needle biopsy specimens and tissue microarrays. *Am J Clin Pathol* 2004; **121**: 220–225.

65. Pisters LL, Pettaway CA, Troncosco P *et al.* Evidence that transfer of functional p53 protein results in increased apoptosis in prostate cancer. *Clin Cancer Res* 2004; **10**: 2587–2593.

66. Cronauer MV, Schulze WA, Burchardt T, Ackermann R, Burchardt M. Inhibition of p53 function diminishes androgen receptor-mediated signaling in prostate cancer cell lines. *Oncogene* 2004; **23**: 3541–3549.

67. Berges RR, Vucanovic J, Epstein JI *et al.* Implication of cell kinetic changes during progression of human prostatic cancer. *Clin Cancer Res* 1995; **1**: 473–480.

68. Dickson RB, McManaway ME, Lippman ME. Estrogen-induced factors of breast cancer cells partially replace estrogen to promote tumor growth. *Science* 1986; **232**: 1540–1543.

69. Goldsworthy TL, Connolly RB, Fransson-Steen R. Apoptosis and cancer risk assessment. *Mutat Res* 1986; **365**: 71–90.

70. Tsujimoto Y, Croce CM. Analysis of the structure, transcripts, and protein products of Bcl-2, the gene involved in human follicular lymphoma. *Proc Natl Acad Sci USA* 1986; **83**: 5214–5218.

71. Vaux D, Cory S, Adams J. Bcl-gene promotes haematopoietic cell survival and co-operates with c-myc to immortalize pre-B cells. *Nature* 1988; **335**: 440–442.

72. Boise LH, Gonzalez-Garcia M, Postema CE *et al.* Bcl-x, a Bcl-2 related gene that functions as a dominant regulator of apoptotic cell death. *Cell* 1993; **74**: 597–608.

73. Krajewski S, Tanaka S. Investigations of the subcellular distribution of the Bcl-2 oncoprotein: residence in the nuclear envelope, endoplasmic reticulum, and outer mitochondrial membranes. *Cancer Res* 1993; **53**: 4701–4714.

74. Reed JC. Bcl-2 and the regulation of programmed cell death. *J Cell Biol* 1994; **124**: 1–6.

75. Reed JC. Prevention of apoptosis as a mechanism of drug resistance. *Haematol Oncol Clin North Am* 1995; **9**: 451–474.

76. Steller H. Mechanisms and genes of cellular suicide. *Science* 1995; **267**: 1445–1449.

77. Hermann JL, Bruckheimer E, McDonnell TJ. Cell death signal transduction and Bcl-2 function. *Biochem Soc Trans* 1996; **24**: 1059–1065.

78. Foster CS, Ke Y. Stem cells in prostatic epithelia. *Int J Exp Pathol* (1997; **78**: 311–329.

79. Hockenbery DM. Bcl-2 protein is topographically restricted to tissues characterized by apoptotic cell death. *Proc Natl Acad Sci USA* 1991; **88**: 6961–6965.

80. Thompson CB. Apoptosis in the pathogenesis and treatment of disease. *Science* 1995; **267**: 1456–1462.

81. Lipponen P, Vesalainen S. Expression of the apoptosis suppressing protein Bcl-2 in prostatic adenocarcinoma is related to tumour malignancy. *Prostate* 1997; **32**: 9–16.

82. Hockenbery D, Zutter M, Hickey W, Nahm M, Korsmeyer SJ. Bcl-2 protein is topographically restricted to tissues characterized by apoptotic cell death. *Proc Natl Acad Sci USA* 1991; **88**: 6961–6965.

83. Colombel M, Symmans G, Gil S *et al.* Detection of the apoptosis-suppressing oncoprotein Bcl-2 in hormone-refractory human prostate cancer. *Am J Pathol* 1993; **143**: 390–400.

84. Colecchia M, Frigo B, Del Boca C *et al.* Detection of apoptosis by the TUNEL technique in clinically localized prostatic cancer before and after combined endocrine therapy. *J Clin Pathol* 1997; **50**: 384–388.

85. McDonnell TJ, Navone NM, Troncosco P *et al.* Expression of Bcl-2 oncoprotein and p53 protein accumulation in bone marrow metastases of androgen independent prostate cancer. *J Urol* 1997; **157**: 569–574.

86. Harari D, Yarden Y. Molecular mechanisms underlying ErbB2/HER2 action in breast cancer. *Oncogene* 2000; **19:** 6102–6114.

87. Yarden Y. Biology of HER2 and its important in breast cancer. *Oncology* 2001; **61:** 1–13.

88. Morris MJ, Reuter VE, Kelly WK *et al*. HER-2 profiling and targeting in prostate carcinoma: A phase II trial of Trastuzumab alone and with Paclitaxel. *Cancer* 2002; **94:** 980–986.

89. Signoretti S, Montironi R, Manola J *et al*. Her-2-neu expression and progression toward androgen independence in human prostate cancer. *J Natl Cancer Inst* 2000; **92:** 1918–1925.

90. Osman I, Scher HI, Drobjnak M *et al*. HER-2/neu (p185neu) protein expression in the natural or treated history of prostate cancer. *Clin Cancer Res* 2001; **7:** 2643–2647.

91. Milarski KL, Welch WJ, Morimoto RI. Cell cycle-dependent association of hsp70 with specific cellular proteins. *J Cell Biol* 1989; **108:** 413–423.

92. Morimoto RI, Tisseres A. *Stress Proteins in Biology and Medicine*. Cold Spring Harbour: Cold Spring Harbour Laboratory Press, 1990.

93. Morimoto RI. Cells in stress: transcriptional activation of heat shock genes. *Science* 1993; **259:** 1409–1410.

94. Tomei LD, Cope FO. *Apoptosis: The Molecular Basis of Cell Death*. Cold Spring Harbour: Cold Spring Harbour Laboratory Press, 1991.

95. Levine AJ, Momand J, Finlay CA. The p53 tumor suppressor gene. *Nature* 1991; **351:** 453–456.

96. Lindquist S, Craig EA. The heat shock proteins. *Annu Rev Genet* (1988; **22:** 631–677.

97. Cornford PA, Evans JD, Dodson AR *et al*. Protein kinase C (PKC) isoenzyme patterns characteristically modulated in early prostate cancer. *Am J Pathol* 1999; **154:** 137–144.

98. Cornford PA, Dodson AR, Parsons KF *et al*. Heat shock protein (HSP) expression independently predicts clinical outcome in prostate cancer. *Cancer Res* 2000; **60:** 7099–7105.

99. Grimes JA, Djamgoz MBA. Electrophysiological characterization of voltage-gated Na$^+$ current expressed in the highly metastatic Mat-LyLu cell line of rat prostate cancer. *J Cell Physiol* 1998; **175:** 50–58.

100. Laniado ME, Lalani EN, Fraser SP *et al*. Expression and functional analysis of voltage-activated Na$^+$ channels in human prostate cancer cell lines and their contribution to invasion *in vitro*. *Am J Pathol* 1997; **150:** 1213–1221.

101. Smith P, Rhodes NP, Shortland AP *et al*. Sodium channel protein expression enhances the invasiveness of rat and human prostate cancer cells. *FEBS Lett* 1998; **423:** 19–24.

102. Schroeder FH, Hop WC, Bloom JH, Mostofi FK. Grading of prostate carcinoma: I. Analysis of the prognostic significance of single characteristics. *Prostate* 1985; **6:** 81–100.

103. Schroeder FH, Hop WC, Bloom JH, Mostofi FK. Grading of prostate carcinoma: multivariant analysis of prognostic parameters. *Prostate* 1985; **7:** 13–20.

104. Wakui S, Furusato M, Itoh T *et al*. Tumor angiogenesis in prostate carcinoma with and without bone marrow metastasis: a morphometric study. *J Pathol* 1992; **168:** 257–262.

105. Fregene T, Khanuja P. Tumor-associated angiogenesis in prostate cancer. *Anticancer Res* 1993; **13:** 2377–2382.

106. Weidner N, Carroll PR, Flax J, Bloomfield W, Folkman J. Tumor angiogenesis correlates with metastasis in invasive prostate carcinoma. *Am J Pathol* 1993; **143:** 401–409.

107. Brawer MK, Deering RE, Brown M, Peterson SD, Bigler SA. Predictors of pathologic stage in prostate cancer. The role of neovascularity. *Cancer* 1994; **73:** 678–687.

108. Hall MC, Zagars GK, Troncoso P *et al*. Significance of tumor angiogenesis in clinically localized prostate carcinoma treated with external beam radiotherapy. *Urology* 1994; **44:** 869–875.

109. Vesalainen S, Lipponen P, Talja M, Alhava E, Syrjanen K. Tumor vascularity and basement membrane structure as prognostic factors in T1-2MO prostatic adenocarcinoma. *Anticancer Res* 1994; **14:** 709–714.

110. Deering RE, Bigler SA, Brown M, Brawer MK. Microvascularity in benign prostatic hyperplasia. *Prostate* 1995; **26:** 111–115.

111. Salamao DR, Graham SD, Bostwick DG. Microvascular invasion in prostate cancer correlates with pathologic stage. *Arch Pathol Lab Med* 1995; **119:** 1050–1054.

112. Barth PJ, Weingartner K, Kohler HH, Bittinger A. Assessment of vascularization in

prostate carcinoma: a morphometric investigation. *Hum Pathol* 1996; **27:** 1306–1310.

113. Bostwick DG, Wheeler TM, Blute M *et al*. Optimized microvessel density analysis improves prediction of cancer stage from prostate needle biopsies. *Urology* 1996; **48:** 47–57.

114. Rogatsch H, Hittmair A, Reissigl A, Mikuz G, Feichtinger H. Microvessel density in core biopsies of prostatic adenocarcinoma: a stage predictor? *J Pathol* 1997; **182:** 205–210.

115. Silberman MA, Partin AW, Veltri RW, Epstein JI. Tumor angiogenesis correlates with progression after radial prostatectomy but not with pathologic stage in Gleason sum 5 to 7 adenocarcinoma of the prostate. *Cancer* 1997; **79:** 772–779.

116. McNeal JE, Yemoto CE. Significance of demonstrable vascular space invasion for the progression of prostatic adenocarcinoma. *Am J Surg Pathol* 1996; **20:** 1351–1360.

117. Gettman MT, Bergstralh EJ, Blute M, Zincke H, Bostwick DG. Prediction of patient outcome in pathologic stage T2 adenocarcinoma of the prostate. Lack of significance for microvessel density analysis. *Urology* 1998; **51:** 79–85.

118. Lissbrant IF, Stattin P, Damber JE, Bergh A. Vascular density is predictor of cancer-specific survival in prostatic carcinoma. *Prostate* 1997; **33:** 38–45.

119. Bahnson RR, Dresner SM, Gooding W, Becich MJ. Incidence and prognostic significance of lymphatic and vascular invasion in radical prostatectomy specimens. *Prostate* 1989; **15:** 149–155.

120. Barraclough R, Savin J, Dube SY, Rudland PS. Molecular cloning and sequence of the gene for p9Ka: a cultured myoepithelial cell protein with strong homology to S-100, a calcium-binding protein. *J Mol Biol* 1987; **198:** 13–20.

121. Goebeler M, Roth J, Van Den Bos C, Ader G, Sorg C. Increase of calcium levels in epithelial cells induces translocation of calcium-binding proteins migration inhibitory factor-related protein 8 (MRP8) and MRP14 to keratin intermediate filaments. *Biochem J* 1995; **309:** 419–424.

122. Jonsson ZO, Hubscher U. Proliferating cell nuclear antigen: more than a clamp for DNA polymerase *Bioessays* 1997; **19:** 967–975.

123. Heiderbrecht HJ, Buck F, Haas K, Wacker HH, Parwaresch R. Monoclonal antibodies Ki-S3 and Ki-S5 yield new data on the 'Ki-67' proteins. *Cell Prolif* 1996; **29:** 413–425.

124. Cher ML, Chew K, Rosenau W, Carroll PR. Cellular proliferation in prostatic adenocarcinoma as assessed by bromodeoxyuridine uptake and Ki-67 and PCNA expression. *Prostate* 1995; **26:** 87–93.

125. Raymond WA, Leong AS, Bolt JW, Milios J, Jose JS. Growth fractions in human prostatic carcinoma determined by Ki-67 immunostaining. *J Pathol* 1988; **156:** 161–167.

126. Giannulis I, Montironi R, Galluzzi CM, de Mictolis M, Diamanti L. Frequency and location of mitoses in prostatic intraepithelial neoplasia (PIN). *Anticancer Res* 1993; **13:** 2447–2451.

127. Montironi R, Magi-Galluzzi C, Muzzonigro G, Prete E, Polito M, Fabris G. Effects of combination endocrine treatment on normal prostate, prostatic intraepithelial neoplasia, and prostatic adenocarcinoma. *J Clin Pathol* 1994; **47:** 906–913.

128. Vesalainen S, Lipponen P, Talja M, Syrjanen K. Mitotic activity and prognosis in prostatic adenocarcinoma. *Prostate* 1995; **26:** 80–86.

129. Gallee MP, Viser-de-Jong E, Ten-Kate FJ, Schroeder FH, Van der Kwast TH. Monoclonal antibody Ki-67 defined growth fraction in benign prostatic hyperplasia and prostate cancer. *J Urol* 1989; **142:** 1342–1346.

130. Chambers TC, McAvoy EM, Jacobs JW, Eilon G. Protein kinase C phosphorylates P-glycoprotein in multidrug resistant human KB carcinoma cells. *J Biol Chem* 1990; **265:** 7679–7686.

131. Svanholm H, Starklint H, Barlebo H, Olsen S. Histological evaluation of prostatic cancer (II): Reproducibility of a histological grading system. *APMIS* 1990; **98:** 229–236.

132. Vesalainen S, Lipponen PK, Talja MT, Alhava EM, Syrjanen KJ. Proliferating cell nuclear antigen and p53 expression as prognostic factors in T1-2MO prostatic adenocarcinoma. *Int J Cancer* 1994; **58:** 303–308.

133. Lipponen P, Vesalainen S, Kasurinen J, Alpa-Opas M, Syrjanen K. A prognostic score for prostatic adenocarcinoma based on clinical, histological biochemical and cytometric data from the primary tumor. *Anticancer Res* 1996; **16:** 2095–2100.

134. van der Voorde WM, Elgamal AA, van Poppel HP, Verbeken EK, Baert L, Lauweryns

JM. Morphologic and immunohistochemical changes in prostate cancer after preoperative hormonal therapy. A comparative study of radical prostatectomies. *Cancer* 1994; **74:** 3164–3175.

135. Kyprianou N, Isaacs J. Expression of transforming growth factor β in the rat ventral prostate during castration-induced programmed cell death. *Mol Endocrinol* 1989; **3:** 1515–1522.

136. Harper ME, Goddard C. Pathological and clinical associations of Ki67 defined growth factors in human prostatic carcinoma. *Prostate* 1992; **20:** 243–253.

137. Brown C, Sauvageot J, Kahane H, Epstein JI. Cell proliferation and apoptosis in prostate cancer – correlation with pathologic stage? *Modern Pathol* 1996; **9:** 205–209.

138. Coetzee LJ, Layfield LJ, Hars V, Paulson DF. Proliferative index determination in prostatic carcinoma tissue: is there any additional prognostic value greater than that of Gleason score, ploidy and pathological stage? *J Urol* 1997; **157:** 214–218.

139. Sadi MV, Barrack ER. Determination of growth fraction in advanced prostate cancer by Ki-67 immunostaining and its relationship to the time to tumor progression after hormonal therapy. *Cancer* 1991; **67:** 3065–3071.

140. Bubendorf L, Sauter G. Ki67 labelling index: an independent predictor of progression in prostate cancer treated by radical prostatectomy. *J Pathol* 1996; **178:** 437–441.

141. Thompson SJ, Mellon K, Charlton RG, Marsh C, Robinson M, Neal DE. p53 and Ki-67 immunoreactivity in human prostate cancer and benign hyperplasia. *Br J Urol* 1992; **69:** 609–613.

142. Moul JW, Bettencourt MC, Sesterhenn IA *et al.* Protein expression of p53, Bcl-2 and Ki-67 (MIB-1) as prognostic biomarkers in patients with surgically treated, clinically localized prostate cancer. *Surgery* 1996; **120:** 159–166.

143. Henke RP, Kruger E, Ayhan N, Hubner D, Hammerer P. Numerical chromosomal aberrations in prostate cancer: correlation with morphology and cell kinetics. *Virchows Arch A* 1993; **422:** 61–66.

144. Aaltoma S, Lipponen P, Vesalainen S, Ala-Opas M, Eskelinen M, Syrjanen K. Value of Ki-67 immunolabelling as a prognostic factor in prostate cancer. *Eur Urol* 1997; **32:** 410–415.

145. Harper ME, Goddard L, Glynne-Jones E *et al.* An immunocytochemical analysis of TGF-alpha expression in benign and malignant prostatic tumors. *Prostate* 1993; **23:** 9–23.

146. Bettencourt MC, Bauer JJ, Sesterhenn IA, Mostofi FK, McLeod DG, Moul JW. Ki-67 expression is a prognostic marker of prostate cancer recurrence after radical prostatectomy. *J Urol* 1996; **156:** 1064–1068.

147. Sadi MV, Walsh PC, Barrack ER. Immunohistochemical study of androgen receptors in metastatic prostate cancer. Comparison of receptor content and response to hormonal therapy. *Cancer* 1991; **67:** 3057–3064.

148. Mashal RD, Lester S, Corless C *et al.* Expression of cell cycle-regulated proteins in prostate cancer. *Cancer Res* 1996; **56:** 4159–4163.

149. McLoughlin J, Foster CS, Price P, WIlliams G, Abel PD. Evaluation of KI-67 monoclonal antibody as prognostic indicator for prostatic carcinoma. *Br J Urol* 1993; **72:** 92–97.

150. Feneley MR, Young MPA, Chinyama C, Kirby RS, Parkinson MC. Ki-67 expression in early prostate cancer and associated pathological lesions. *J Clin Pathol* 1996; **49:** 741–748.

151. Speights VOJ, Arber DA, Riggs MW, Arber J, Chen PY. Proliferative index of organ-confined prostatic adenocarcinoma determined by MIB-1. *J Urol Pathol* 1996; **4:** 25–30.

152. Scalzo DA, Kallakury BVS, Gaddipati RV *et al.* Cell proliferation rate by MIB-1 immunohistochemistry predicts postradiation recurrence in prostatic adenocarcinoma. *Am J Clin Pathol* 1997; **109:** 163–168.

153. Montironi R, Magi-Galluzzi C, Fabris G. Apoptotic bodies in prostatic intraepithelial neoplasia and prostatic adenocarcinoma following total androgen ablation. *Pathol Res Pract* 1995; **191:** 873–880.

154. Kyprianou N, Tu H, Jacobs SC. Apoptotic versus proliferative activities in human benign prostatic hyperplasia. *Hum Pathol* 1996; **27:** 668–675.

155. Tang DG, Porter AT. Target to apoptosis: a hopeful weapon for prostate cancer. *Prostate* 1997; **32:** 284–293.

156. Wheeler TM, Rogers E, Aihara M, Scardino PT, Thompson TC. Apoptotic index as a biomarker in prostatic intraepithelial neoplasia (PIN) and prostate cancer. *J Cell Biochem* 1994; **19:** 202–207.

157. Aihara M, Scardino PT, Truong LD *et al*. The frequency of apoptosis correlates with the prognosis of Gleason Grade 3 adenocarcinoma of the prostate. *Cancer* 1995; **75**: 522–529.

158. Drachenberg CB, Ioffe OB, Papadimitriou JC. Progressive increase of apoptosis in prostatic intraepithelial neoplasia and carcinoma. *Arch Pathol Lab Med* 1997; **121**: 54–58.

159. Yang E, Korsmeyer SJ. Molecular thanatopsis: a discourse on the Bcl-2 family and cell death. *Blood* 1996; **88**: 386–401.

160. Hasson MO, Maksem J. The prostatic perineural space and its relation to tumor spread. An ultrastructural study. *Am J Surg Pathol* 1980; **4**: 143–148.

161. Korsmeyer SJ. Bcl-2: an antidote to programmed cell death. *Cancer Surveys* 1992; **15**: 105–118.

162. Westin P, Stattin P, Damber JE, Bergh A. Castration therapy rapidly induces apoptosis in a minority and decreases cell proliferation in a majority of human tumours. *Am J Pathol* 1995; **146**: 1368–1375.

163. Djakiew D. Role of nerve growth factor-like protein in the paracrine regulation of prostate growth. *J Androl* 1992; **13**: 476–487.

164. Di Sant'Agnese PA, de Mesy Jensen KL, Churukian CL, Agarwal MM. Human prostatic endocrine-paracrine (APUD) cells. *Arch Pathol Lab Med* 1985; **109**: 607–612.

165. Kimura N, Hoshi S, Takahashi M, Shizawa S, Nagura H. Plasma chromogranin A in prostatic carcinoma and neuroendocrine cancers. *J Urol* 1997; **157**: 565–568.

166. Debes JD, Tindall DJ. Mechanisms of androgen-refractory prostate cancer. *N Engl J Med* 2004; **351**: 1488–1490.

167. Di Sant'Agnese PA, Cockett AT. The prostatic endocrine-paracrine (neuroendocrine) regulatory system and neuroendocrine differentiation in prostatic carcinoma: a review and future directions in basic research. *J Urol* 1994; **152**: 1927–1931.

168. van de Voorde WM, Van Poppel HP, Verbeken EK, Oyen RH, Baert LV, Lauweryns JM. Morphologic and neuroendocrine features of adenocarcinoma arising in the transition zone and in the peripheral zone of the prostate. *Modern Pathol* 1995; **8**: 91–98.

169. Weistein MH, Partin AW, Veltri RW, Epstein JI. Neuroendocrine differentiation in prostate cancer: enhanced prediction of progression after radical prostatectomy. *Hum Pathol* 1996; **27**: 683–687.

170. Abrahamsson PA, Falkner S, Falt K, Girmelius L. The course of neuroendocrine differentiation in prostatic carcinomas. An immunohistochemical study testing chromogranin A as an 'endocrine marker'. *Pathol Res Pract* 1989; **185**: 373–380.

171. Di Sant'Agnese PA. Neuroendocrine differentiation in carcinoma of the prostate. Diagnosis, prognostic and therapeutic implications. *Cancer* 1992; **70**: 254–268.

172. Deftos LJ, Nakada S, Burton DW, Di Sant'Agnese PA, Cockett AT, Abrahamsson PA. Immunoassay and immunohistology studies of chromogranin A as a neuroendocrine marker in patients with carcinoma of the prostate. *Urology* 1996; **48**: 58–62.

173. Noordzij MA, van der Kwast TH, van Steenbrugge A, Hop WJ, Schroder FH. The prognostic influence of neuroendocrine cells in prostate cancer: results of a long-term follow-up study with patients treated by radical prostatectomy. *Int J Cancer* 1995; **62**: 252–258.

174. Cohen P, Peehl DM, Baker B, Liu F, Hintz RL, Rosenfeld RG. Insulin-like growth factor axis abnormalities in prostatic stromal cells from patients with benign prostatic hyperplasia. *J Clin Endocrinol Metab* 1994; **79**: 1410–1415.

175. Aprikian AG, Cordon-Cardo C, Fair WR *et al*. Neuroendocrine differentiation in metastatic prostatic adenocarcinoma. *J Urol* 1994; **151**: 914–919.

176. Speights VO, Cohen MK, Riggs MW, Coffield KS, Keegan G, Arber DA. Neuroendocrine stains and proliferative indices of prostatic adenocarcinomas in transurethral resection samples. *Br J Urol* 1997; **80**: 281–186.

177. Hakima JM, Rondinelli RH, Schoenberg MP, Barrack ER. Androgen-receptor gene structure and function in prostate cancer. *World J Urol* 1996; **14**: 329–337.

178. Chodak GW, Kranc DM, Puy LA, Takeda H, Johnson K, Chang C. Nuclear localization of androgen receptor in heterogeneous samples of normal, hyperplastic and neoplastic human prostate. *J Urol* 1992; **147**: 798–803.

179. Sadi M, Barrack ER. Image analysis of androgen receptor immunostaining in metastatic prostate cancer. Heterogeneity as a predictor of response to hormonal therapy. *Cancer* 1993; **71**: 2574–2580.

180. Tilley WD, Lim-Tio SS, Horsfall DJ, Aspinall JO, Marshall VR, Skinner JM. Detection of discrete androgen receptor epitopes in prostate cancer by immunostaining: measurement by color video image analysis. *Cancer Res* 1994; **54:** 4096–4102.

181. Foster CS, Falconer A, Dodson AR *et al.* Transcription factor E2F3 overexpressed in prostate cancer independently predicts clinical outcome. *Oncogene* 2004; **23:** 5871–5879.

182. Bashir I, Sikora K, Foster CS. Multidrug resistance and behavioral phenotype of cancer cells. *Cell Biol Int* 1993; **17:** 907–917.

183. Ciocca DR, Clark GM, Tandon AK, Fuqua SAN, Welch WJ, McGuire WL. Heat shock protein hsp70 in patients with axillary lymph node-negative breast cancer: prognostic implications. *J Natl Cancer Inst* 1993; **85:** 570–574.

184. Cattoretti G, Becker MHG, Key G *et al.* Monoclonal antibodies against recombinant parts of Ki-67 antigen (MIB-1) and (MIB-3) detect proliferating cells in microwave processed formalin-fixed paraffin sections. *J Pathol* 1992; **168:** 357–360.

185. Glynne-Jones E, Goddard L, Harper ME. Comparative analysis of mRNA and protein expression for epidermal growth factor receptor and ligands relative to the proliferation index in human prostate tissue. *Hum Pathol* 1996; **27:** 688–694.

Index

137